Medical
& Surgical
Emergencies

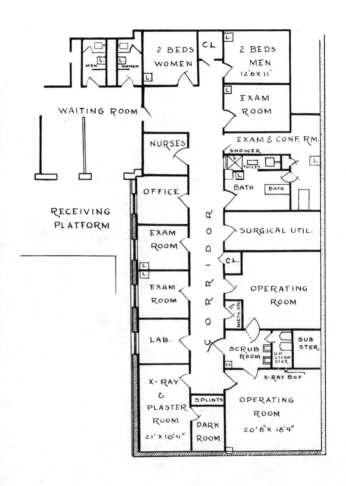

Representative Floor Plan of a Typical Emergency Service

MEDICAL & SURGICAL EMERGENCIES

Edited by
JOHN H. SCHNEEWIND, M.D. (Deceased)
Professor of Surgery and Chief of Emergency Service
University of Illinois Hospitals

THIRD EDITION

YEAR BOOK MEDICAL PUBLISHERS, INC.
35 East Wacker Drive / Chicago

Reprinted, January 1966
Second Edition, 1968
Reprinted, April 1970
Third Edition, 1973

Library of Congress Catalog Card Number: 72-93719
International Standard Book Number: 0-8151-7559-0

Cover photograph courtesy of Merck Sharp & Dohme.

Publisher's Note

Only two weeks after delivering the final materials for the third edition of the manual *Medical and Surgical Emergencies,* that he had edited so ably since 1963, Dr. John H. Schneewind passed away. As in earlier editions, the manuscript that Dr. Schneewind prepared was very carefully organized and well written, and we are grateful to all of his collaborators for their fine cooperation in the preparation of their material.

The burden of answering our queries and other duties that an editor may be called upon to assume during the publisher's preparation of his manuscript for press have been graciously undertaken by Dr. Lloyd Nyhus, Chairman of Surgery, Abraham Lincoln School of Medicine. We are indeed grateful to him for offering his help immediately upon the death of Dr. Schneewind, who will be sorely missed as the editor and originator of this ever-popular manual.

Preface to the Third Edition

Ten new chapters have been added to the Third Edition
of *Medical and Surgical Emergencies*. These are:

> Antibiotics in the Emergency Room
> Cardiopulmonary Resuscitation
> Emergency Care of Acute Myocardial Infarction
> Adult Regional Anesthesia
> Tetanus and Rabies
> Emergencies of the Respiratory System
> Peripheral Vascular Emergencies
> Management of Convulsive Disorders
> Pediatric Anesthesia in the Emergency Service
> Proctologic Emergencies.

In addition, almost every other chapter has been completely revised. The format has been changed to more of an
outline form for easy readability and quick reference.

Again, we are indebted to the members of our faculty as
well as the other authors for their contributions. A word of
thanks is due to Robert J. Baker, M.D., for going over the
chapter on Cardiopulmonary Resuscitation with Dr. Boyd.
We are also greatly indebted to Mr. William R. Schwarz, who
has done all of the drawings and, finally, to Lloyd M. Nyhus,
M.D., Professor and Head, Department of Surgery, who has
made it possible to complete this revision.

Preface to the First Edition

This manual was designed originally for use at the University of Illinois Hospitals and was privately printed and distributed through two editions for that purpose. The present volume has been broadened as much as possible so that it might be of value to hospitals which are not university affiliated and which have no interns or residents. This has been accomplished by the addition of new sections on Resuscitation and Anesthesia, Medical Emergencies. Emergencies in Otolaryngology and Ocular Emergencies. Many of the original sections have been revised, including those on Pediatrics, Poisons, Fractures, and so on, and illustrations have been added in appropriate places. Also new is Part III, Preparation for Disaster.

Some subjects, such as cardiac arrest, are discussed in more than one section, but the management is essentially similar. We realize that many controversial points of therapy are presented without extensive discussion, but believe that this is unavoidable in a manual of this kind.

The editor expresses his indebtedness to the faculty members whose contributions made this manual possible.

John H. Schneewind

Table of Contents

PART I

GENERAL CONSIDERATIONS

General Rules

JOHN H. SCHNEEWIND, M.D.

1. PRECAUTIONS IN ASEPSIS

A cap and mask should be worn at all times when examining open wounds or burns.

2. MAGNITUDE

A. Unless a life or death situation, all operations will be scheduled as emergencies in the Main Operating Suite.
B. Minor lacerations are the only exceptions.

3. CONSENT FOR TREATMENT

A. *Written consent must* be obtained prior to any treatment in the Emergency Service.
B. If an unusual or major procedure is required immediately, use the regular hospital operative permit and attach to the records.
C. In all instances when written permission is unobtainable, the chief of the Emergency Service, the surgeon in charge or the medical director must be notified and the problem discussed with him.
D. When a lifesaving emergency operation, such as a tracheostomy or thoracostomy, is necessary, permission is desirable but must not delay treatment.
E. Consent by a guardian or a relative is very desirable but not mandatory if a senior attending surgeon, administrator or senior surgical resident concurs.

3

4. TETANUS PROPHYLAXIS

A. Tetanus toxoid usually is given to patients who enter the Emergency Service for treatment of a soft-tissue wound. Chapter 7, "Tetanus and Rabies," should be used as a guide for treatment.

B. A record of the amount and type of drug given *must* be made on the Emergency Service record.

5. SKULL ROENTGENOGRAMS

A. Patients with head injuries caused by a blow or who have been unconscious must be observed until it is certain that they have not sustained cerebral or other damage.

B. Such patients should have skull and cervical spine x-ray films and an *official report* from the Radiology Department prior to discharge.

C. Patients with simple scalp lacerations need not have skull films unless there is a possibility of a fracture.

D. If in doubt as to the severity of the injury, keep the patient under observation until he is stable and obviously well enough to go home.

E. He should be accompanied by a relative.

F. Follow-up examinations should be frequent.

G. If in doubt, *hospitalize!*

6. THE ALCOHOLIC PATIENT

A. Statements written in the medical record should describe the patient as "having the odor of alcohol, etc."

B. *Do not write:* "The patient was drunk." *or* "The patient was intoxicated."

C. Do not make the mistake of overlooking an acute illness or injury.

7. NARCOTICS

A. Narcotics are not given to patients who are scheduled to leave the Emergency Service without admission to the hospital.

B. Oral codeine in doses not to exceed 60 mg. every 4 hours, if needed, may be prescribed or dispensed for periods of 24-48 hours.

C. The drug is *not* given until the patient arrives at home unless accompanied by a relative or friend.

8. FOLLOW-UP CARE

A. The patient should be referred for continuing care to his family physician, who should be notified of the findings and treatment rendered.

B. If the patient has no physician, he should be given a list from which to choose.

C. He must be given *written instructions* regarding subsequent care and a *definite written* appointment for follow-up care by his physician or the appropriate out-patient facility.

9. DEATH CASES

If a patient is dead or dies shortly after arrival, the coroner must be notified *at once*.

10. POLICE NOTIFICATION

A. The police must be notified immediately of all gunshot wounds, stabbings, assaults, accidents, rapes, attempted suicides, poisonings, drug addiction, animal bites, as well as cases in which there is some suspicion of foul play.

B. If a suspect "battered child" is brought in, follow the procedures outlined in Chapter 19, "Pediatric Medical Emergencies."

11. HEALTH DEPARTMENT NOTIFICATION

Communicable diseases, animal bites and poisonings should be reported to the Health Department.

12. INFORMATION CONCERNING PATIENTS

Basic information, i.e., sociologic information, nature of the accident and general information as to the type

of injury and condition of the patient may be released to press, radio and television.

13. UNUSUAL OCCURRENCE REPORTS

Any incidents in this category should be covered by a
detailed report and notes in the *Emergency Service
record.*

14. CUSTODY CASES

A. If the patient is brought to the Emergency Service
   with established or suspected injuries that would
   be affected adversely by transfer to another institution, the medical needs of the patient are para-
   mount.
B. Other factors, such as medicolegal implications,
   problems of disposition, police custody, etc., *must
   not* be allowed to influence judgment when deciding upon proper treatment and hospitalization!
C. If it is necessary to maintain the patient under
   guard, this responsibility will be assumed by the
   police or the law enforcement agency concerned.

"Ten Commandments"

JOHN H. SCHNEEWIND, M.D.

1. **DO FIRST THINGS FIRST.**

   When a seriously injured patient arrives, check the following at once:
   A. IS PATIENT BREATHING?
      CLEAR AIRWAY. INTUBATE PATIENT WITH AN ENDOTRACHEAL TUBE, IF NEEDED.
   B. IS PATIENT BLEEDING?
      IF SO, APPLY A PRESSURE DRESSING.
   C. TREAT FOR SHOCK.
   D. START CARDIOPULMONARY RESUSCITATION IMMEDIATELY IF NEEDED (CHAP. 1).

2. **WRITTEN CONSENT MUST BE OBTAINED PRIOR TO TREATMENT IN A GENUINE LIFE OR DEATH SITUATION. PERMISSION BY THE CLOSEST RELATIVE IS VERY DESIRABLE BUT SHOULD NOT DELAY TREATMENT.**

3. **PATIENTS WITH HEAD INJURIES REQUIRE EXPERT CARE** (CHAP. 11).

   These patients must be observed until—
   A. It is certain that no cerebrospinal or other injury is present.
   B. Skull and cervical spine roentgenograms reveal no fracture. Treat the *patient*—not the x-ray film.

4. **INFANTS AND CHILDREN SHOULD BE HOSPITALIZED**—if suffering from—
   A. Temperature of 104° F. or over.

    B. Convulsions.
    C. Poisons.
    D. Head injuries.
    E. Stridor and dyspnea.
    F. Full-thickness or partial-thickness burns of 10% body area or more (see Chap. 13).

5. **ALCOHOLICS MAY BE SERIOUSLY INJURED OR ACUTELY ILL!**

   Do not overlook a skull fracture, diabetic coma, etc., in an alcoholic.

6. **HUMAN BITE WOUNDS ARE SERIOUS.** See Chapter 5. "Injuries and Infections of the Hand."

   A. Never suture the wound primarily.
   B. The patient should be hospitalized.

7. **REMEMBER TETANUS PROPHYLAXIS.** See Chapter 7, "Tetanus and Rabies."

8. **ALWAYS CALL FOR HELP IF SEVERAL SERIOUSLY ILL OR INJURED PATIENTS ARE BROUGHT IN SIMULTANEOUSLY.**

9. **DO NOT HESITATE TO OBSERVE BORDERLINE PATIENTS.**

10. **ADVICE AND CONSULTATION ARE ALWAYS AVAILABLE. IF IN ANY DOUBT, CALL!**

The Acutely Ill or Injured Patient

JOHN H. SCHNEEWIND, M.D.

I. GENERAL CONSIDERATIONS

A. Minimal and gentle handling is axiomatic in treating acutely ill or injured patients.

B. This is especially true during the initial examination. A superficial injury may distract attention from a fractured cervical spine or a lacerated spleen.

C. Injudicious movement may accentuate shock, stir up quiescent hemorrhage or cause severe spinal cord damage.

D. The unconscious patient may present a difficult problem. Accurate diagnosis and immediate treatment may save his life.

E. "First things first" is another axiom which must be observed.
   1. The cleansing and dressing of a patient with severe burns prior to institution of treatment of burn shock may spell disaster.
   2. Treatment of obvious fractures while active intra-abdominal hemorrhage proceeds undetected is not uncommon.

F. It may be helpful to classify some conditions which can produce loss of consciousness and sensorial dysfunction.

   1. **Circulatory Shock** (see Chap. 1).
      a. Hemorrhage.
      b. Trauma.
      c. Burns.

9

    d. Exposure.
    e. Myocardial infarction.
    f. Heart failure.
    g. Cardiac tamponade.

2. **Intracranial Lesions** (see Chap. 11).
    a. Trauma.
    b. Stroke.
    c. Vascular spasm.
    d. Embolism.
    e. Tumors.
    f. Infection.

3. **Physiochemical Coma.**

The following group is concerned with the effects of deranged *intrinsic* physiology or *extrinsic* poisons.
    a. Alcoholism.
    b. Poisons.
    c. Diabetic coma.
    d. Insulin shock.
    e. Uremia.
    f. Dehydration and electrolytic depletion.
    g. Toxemia.
    h. Psychoses.

II. PHYSICAL EXAMINATION

It is essential that the Emergency Service physician master the technique of a rapid, thorough examination of the acutely ill patient. It is surprising how much information can be obtained by a systematic approach.

A. INITIAL INSPECTION

In the initial inspection, the examiner should look for evidence of severe illness or injury which may require immediate attention. Of crucial importance:

1. *Is the Patient Breathing?*
    a. The examiner must be sure that the tongue is forward and that vomitus, mucus or blood is not blocking the airway.

    b. An endotracheal tube should be inserted if necessary.

2. *Is the Patient Bleeding?*
   a. Severe wounds require immediate attention when there is acute bleeding.
   b. The bleeding must be controlled by a pressure dressing.
   c. Occasionally, TEMPORARY application of a tourniquet is indicated.
   d. If so, it must be *released every 10 minutes* for a short period.

3. *Is the Patient in Shock?*
   a. Intravenous administration of fluids such as dextran, plasma or whole blood is required.

4. *Is there a Fracture Deformity?*
   a. Inspection may reveal swelling, ecchymosis or an obvious deformity.
   b. Point tenderness, false motion, crepitus, bony irregularity and loss of function are other signs.
   c. Multiple rib fractures may be associated with intrathoracic injury.

5. *Is the Sensorium Affected?*
   a. Loss of consciousness may be due to pre-existing disease or intracranial trauma.
   b. The state of consciousness is often an index of the seriousness of the illness or injury.

B. HISTORY

1. A rapid, brief history of the accident or illness should be obtained from the patient by direct questioning if he is able to respond coherently.
2. It may be necessary to obtain the information from a witness to the accident or from a member of the family.
3. Important points which must be established are:
   a. State of consciousness *prior to* and *following* injury or illness.

   b. Pre-existing disease or disability.
   c. Previous treatment rendered, especially adminis-
       tration of narcotics.

C. EXAMINATION

The physician should now do a rapid, thorough examination, with some idea of what he may encounter and what
aspects of the examination must be done with extreme
care.

Antibiotics in the Emergency Service

LOUISE RIFF, M.D.

I. GENERAL PRINCIPLES

A. Sound judgment is required in order to approve the use of antibiotics on an outpatient basis when a serious infection is possible. Follow-up therapy may be inadequate, and symptomatic improvement without cure is to the patient's detriment.

   Axiom: If a wound or disease state is severe enough to require antibiotics, hospitalization should be considered carefully!

B. *Prophylactic use of antibiotics* has virtually no place in the Emergency Service.

   1. *Exceptions:*
      a. Human bites.
      b. Gonococcus (GC) exposure.
      c. Pharyngitis in patients with rheumatic heart disease.

   2. Any time *any* antimicrobial is used, significant alteration of the body flora and the emergence of resistant strains can occur.

   3. The cost is high, the spectrum limited and the danger of adverse reactions is possible.

C. It is *absolutely essential* that *an adequate past history of allergy and drug reaction be obtained* from every patient who is to receive antibiotics.

D. If an antimicrobial agent is to be used, the specific organisms *must* be known or presumed on good evidence.

13

1. *Gram stain* is invaluable in establishing the *general class* of the organism. It is extremely helpful—
   a. If cultures are lost.
   b. If culture and sensitivities are *inconsistent* with the clinical course of the patient.
   c. If a lethal organism is present.
   d. If the antibiotics used may change the flora.
   e. Examples are:
      1) Anaerobic bacteria cultured as aerobes.
      2) Encapsulated Klebsiella in the sputum.
      3) Clostridia in a wound.
2. Specimens of the exudate *must* be sent for *culture and sensitivity* in *every* infection. If an anaerobe is suspected, the appropriate media should be used.

II. UPPER RESPIRATORY INFECTIONS

A. The antibiotic therapy of *acute pharyngitis, tonsillitis* and *sinusitis* is properly prescribed only when cultures of nose, throat, and nasopharynx are taken or known. Remember that in those people seeking emergency aid, less than 50% of pharyngitis and less than 5% of laryngitis are bacterial.

B. Supportive therapy with antipyretics, antihistamines, and antitussives will often suffice until the culture results are available. If specific therapy is started without culture results, one must justify the cost (even of penicillin) and the possibility of the patient with group A beta strep being inadequately treated. Patients may fail follow-up visits if they are symptomatically improved.

C. *Group A beta hemolytic streptococcal infections* require penicillin therapy for 10 days. (See section on Penicillin; check for allergy.) Adults should be given:

1. *Procaine penicillin,* 600,000 units I.M. daily for 10 days.
2. *Procaine penicillin* with aluminum monostearate in oil, 600,000 units I.M. every *third* day for 3 doses.

3. *Phenoxymethyl penicillin* (PCN-VK) 250 mg. t.i.d. orally for at least 10 days.
4. *Benzathine penicillin,* 1,200,000 units. This is the least desirable.
5. *Erythromycin or lincomycin,* in a dosage of 250 mg. q.i.d. for adults may be substituted for penicillin if necessary.

D. **OTITIS MEDIA** (see Chap. 19).

1. Cultures should be taken. In children under the age of 6 years, Hemophilus influenzae is a common cause of otitis media.
2. Ampicillin, 25 mg./kg./day in 4 divided doses for 7 days may be prescribed.
3. Over age 6, pneumococci or non-group A beta strep are the most likely causes; phenoxymethyl penicillin, 25 mg./kg./day for 7 days is adequate. (See section on Penicillin; check for allergy.)

III. LOWER RESPIRATORY INFECTION

A. BRONCHITIS AND PNEUMONIA

1. The exacerbation of chronic bronchitis or acute purulent bronchitis often can be adequately treated. The danger is in missing the presence of pneumonia.
2. *Adequate examination of the chest and a chest x-ray film are required.*
3. A *gram* stain is mandatory. If pus cells with intracellular organisms are present and the daily volume of sputum and its purulence have both increased, therapy should be instituted.
4. Predominant *gram-negative* organisms must be evaluated very carefully.
5. *There is no role for outpatient therapy of pneumonia,* diplococcal or any other type. There still remains a significant morbidity and mortality with pneumonia—early death, incomplete resolution, empyema and sepsis are all possible.

B. TREATMENT

   1. **Tetracycline**

      a. Chronic bronchitis or acute purulent bronchitis can often be adequately treated with tetracycline HCl, 15-30 mg./kg. in 4 divided doses (250-500 mg. q.i.d. for adults). It should *not* be prescribed for pregnant women.

      b. All tetracyclines significantly alter the body flora with the resulting possibility of superinfection with more pathogenic organisms than the original flora. G.I. upset is the most common side effect. Tetracycline HCl is excreted primarily by the kidney. Patients with normal renal function may develop an elevated Blood Urea Nitrogen (BUN).

      c. Tetracyclines should not be used in people with known impairment of renal function. Significant alteration of hepatic and/or renal function necessitates reconsideration of the use of these drugs.

   2. **Ampicillin** may be substituted if contraindications to tetracycline are present.

IV. SKIN

See Chapter 5, "Injuries and Infections of the Hand."

A. When *cellulitis* is the problem, a culture can be obtained by first preparing the skin with iodine and alcohol, then injecting 1 ml. of sterile saline near the spreading edge, quickly followed by aspiration. The aspirate is placed in a blood culture bottle. Since streptococci are the most frequent cause of this lesion, penicillin therapy may be indicated.

B. *Lacerations and puncture* wounds require thorough cleaning as primary therapy and antimicrobials *only* as the extent of the wound and gram stain, culture, and sensitivities indicate.

C. In a wound demonstrating erythema, swelling, pain and *pus,* a gram stain, culture and sensitivities offer the best evidence for initial treatment.

D. *Human bites* should be treated with procaine penicillin, 600,000 units daily for 3 days (adult dose). Initial thorough local cleaning and daily inspection are important.

V. PELVIC INFLAMMATORY DISEASE

See Chapter 15, "Obstetrical and Gynecological Emergencies."

A. Pelvic inflammatory disease frequently is due to gonococci (GC); however, the endogenous vaginal flora, which commonly include enterococci, E. coli and bacteroides, can be involved.

B. The danger of diagnosing P.I.D. instead of ruptured ectopic pregnancy or other gynecologic emergency must be kept in mind. In addition, patients with P.I.D. have a higher frequency of associated gynecologic problems.

C. Cultures are made by stripping the urethra, scraping the cervical os and probing the rectum.

D. These cultures should be plated immediately on Thayer Martin or chocolate agar media for incubation under CO_2 (for GC), as well as on routine media.

E. The recommended *THERAPY* for GC in females is 4.8 million units of aqueous procaine penicillin (2.4 million each buttock) *plus* probenecid. A 500-mg dose of probenecid should be given 1/2 hour before the penicillin, and 6, 12 and 18 hours afterwards. Therapy is the same for males.

Spectinomycin, an aminocyclitol antibiotic, achieves comparable results, but is expensive. It is given in an I.M. dose of 2 and 4 Gm. to males and females, respectively. Spectinomycin is licensed only for the treatment of GC and no other diseases. Urticaria has been noted in about 0.5% of patients.

An *oral* alternative is tetracycline, 1.5 Gm. immediately, followed by 500 mg. twice daily for 4 days (total dose, 9 Gm.), but it is of secondary worth.

N.B. Recommendations for the treatment of gonorrhea are difficult to formulate because of continuously developing resistance and the different geographic distribution of resistance. *It must be remembered that single dose treatment may not be curative.*

VI. URINARY TRACT INFECTION

See Chapter 16, "Management of Urological Problems."

A. Emergency Service treatment of mild, acute urinary tract infection may be effective *if* symptoms are confined to the lower urinary tract, and the patient does not have a history of chronic infection.

B. Obtain clean-voided, midstream urine for culture and sensitivity. Once results are known, therapy may be changed if necessary.

C. Cultures of the urine during therapy, if sterile, will insure that an adequate drug in sufficient dosage is being given. With an effective agent, the urine should be sterile after 48 hours of therapy.

D. Treatment should continue for 7 days. A follow-up culture *1 month* after therapy is important, as symptoms may disappear while bacteria persist.

E. Patients with acute urinary tract symptoms who have a past history of *repeated or chronic infections* should not be treated primarily from the Emergency Service. They are likely to have resistant organisms, complications or both.

Cultures should be taken, and the patient should be referred promptly for definitive therapy or hospitalized. Sepsis is a real danger in patients with repeated, complicated urinary tract infections.

F. A patient with *flank pain or tenderness,* indicating upper urinary tract infection, must be evaluated carefully before making a decision to treat from the Emergency Service.
1. If fever is absent or low-grade, check to be sure the patient has not recently taken aspirin.

2. Significant fever or additional symptoms such as vomiting are strong considerations for hospitalization.
3. A history of one or more shaking chills is usually an indication of bacteremia.

G. **Treatment**

Sulfonamides. The most inexpensive, easily administered and drug of choice for an *acute urinary tract infection* in a patient not chronically afflicted is a sulfonamide. Sulfisoxazole, in dosages of 1-2 Gm. 4 times daily (100-150 mg./kg./day, preceded by a loading dose of 4 Gm. is adequate.
1. Instruct the patient to maintain a high fluid intake.
2. Resistance develops rapidly and the sulfas are of little use for chronic infections.
3. Therapy should be continued for 2 weeks. Check for allergies.
4. Adequate *follow-up* is necessary, for this is an extremely common infection (second only to respiratory infections), and persistent infection is possible without the presence of symptoms.

VII. PENICILLIN

A. This antibiotic is excreted by the kidney and may be used in a wide range of clinical infections.
1. It is therapeutic for group A beta hemolytic streptococci, which usually are susceptible to 0.01 mcg./ml. (1 unit = 0.63 mcg./ml.), and can kill most strains of pneumococci, gonococci and meningococci if proper dosage and duration of therapy are used.

B. **ADVERSE REACTIONS**

See Chapter 25, "Allergic Emergencies."

1. The toxicity and hypersensitivity responses associated with this drug range from pain at injection to anaphylaxis and death.

2. Fever, eosinophilia, leukopenia, Coombs'-positive hemolytic anemia and nephritis all have been reported.
3. Allergic reactions occur in 2.5-15% of patients, depending on the mode of data collection.
4. Allergic reactions have been documented in people denying past exposure to penicillin. Reactions are more frequent in people with a history of atopy and in adults rather than children.
5. Only 0.1% of all penicillin reactions cause anaphylaxis, but the mortality with this group ranges from 10-25%.

C. IMMUNOLOGIC REACTIONS

1. Immunologic reactions are generally categorized into *reagin-mediated* reactions and those correlated with IgM and IgG.
2. The immediate, or anaphylactic, and the accelerated, or urticarial, reactions are *reagin-mediated*.
3. Examples of IgM- and IgG-correlated reactions are Coombs'-positive (red cell agglutination), hemolytic anemia and the rare case of agranulocytopenia from penicillin.
4. Data have shown that about 15% are accelerated reactions, 50% are late urticarial or exanthemas and 20% are uncertain.
5. Benzyl penicilloyl polylysine (BPL) and minor determinant mixtures (MDM) are substances with which patients can be tested for their reaction to penicillin. They are *specific* for penicillin. These tests allow identification of the patient with a potential immediate or accelerated reaction.
6. The indications for skin testing are also indications for *consultation*. Potentially disastrous reactions have occurred during the skin-testing procedure itself:

D. PREPARATIONS

1. *Benzyl Penicillin (PCN.G)* is susceptible to penicillinase and inactivated by gastric acid. The G.I. absorption of oral preparations is variable.
2. *Procaine PCN G* for I.M. injection gives detectable blood levels for *12-24* hours.
3. *Procaine PCN G in aluminum monostearate* for I.M. injection gives detectable blood levels for *48-72* hours.
4. *Benzathine PCN G (Bicillin)* for I.M. injection only; 1.2 million units gives detectable blood levels for *3-4 weeks.*
5. *Phenoxymethyl PCN (Pen V) and Phenoxyethyl PCN (phenethicillin)* are similar to PCN G in antibacterial activity but are acid-stable and well absorbed.
   a. Each 125 mg. of the drug equals 200,000 units.
   b. Because the absorption of both of these preparations may be *enhanced* by the presence of food in the stomach, they should be taken *before* or *after* meals.

E. AMPICILLIN

1. Ampicillin is acid-stable but *not* penicillinase-resistant.
2. It is well absorbed after oral administration.
3. It is *less* active than PCN G against common gram-positive cocci.
4. Adverse reactions are similar to those produced by PCN G; skin reactions are more frequent than with PCN G.
5. G.I. disturbance, superinfections, and cross-sensitivity reactions occur.

PART II

DIAGNOSIS and TREATMENT

CHAPTER 1

Cardiopulmonary Resuscitation

DAVID R. BOYD, M.D.C.M.

I. GENERAL CONSIDERATIONS

A. Unexpected and irreversible failure of ventilation and circulation may be caused by acute myocardial infarction, anaphylactic and drug reactions, asphyxia, electric shock and drowning. They are catastrophes that demand immediate and proper systematic treatment.

B. Complete cerebral anoxia over 4 minutes will cause permanent damage and beyond 6-8 minutes will cause death.

C. Cessation of normal circulation causes rapid cyclic deterioration which is characterized by hypoxia, lactic acidosis and hypercarbia. Pre-existing heart disease, electrolyte imbalance, medication or anesthetics may precipitate this collapse.

D. Not well understood are the reflex vagus-induced arrests secondary to stimulation of the esophagus and tracheobronchial tree; similar arrest may occur during rectal and proctoscopic examination.

E. Preanesthetic doses of atropine may have worn off by the end of a long (4-hour) operation and may make the patient more susceptible to the complication in D, above.

F. Electrolyte imbalance, mainly hyperkalemia either from endogenous or exogenous sources, is of prime importance. The ratio of ionized serum calcium to potassium and their antagonistic actions on the myocardium are important during massive transfusion of banked blood. It is high in potassium as well as calcium-binding citrate.

G. Other causes of cardiac arrest include: pulmonary emboli, electrocution or any cause of hypoxia.

H. Primary ventilatory failure is caused by hypoxia, central nervous system or spinal cord trauma and respiratory depression from narcotics.

II. MANAGEMENT OF CARDIOPULMONARY ARREST

This is best understood by defining the measures that must be initiated as soon as the diagnosis is established and which are necessary to sustain and support cardiopulmonary function.

A. EMERGENCY MEASURES (*A* for Airway)

1. Begin treatment if there is no obtainable blood pressure or pulse for *10 seconds.*
2. Place patient in *supine* position on a hard surface (metal or plastic tray *under* the chest).
3. Establish a *clear airway*.
    a. Clean out mouth and pharynx (manually or by suction).
    b. Tilt head back and pull chin forward.
    c. Insert an oropharyngeal airway or endotracheal tube, if necessary.

B. ESTABLISH VENTILATION (*B* for Breathing)

1. **Mouth-to-mouth.** A handkerchief may be interposed between the operator's mouth and patient.
2. Use "Ambu" bag and mask if available.
3. Provide an adequate tidal volume. Note extent of chest excursion. Optimal rates are:
    a. Adults—12 times per minute.
    b. Children—20 times per minute.
    c. Infants—30 times per minute.
    d. Ventilate *adults* until chest expands to beyond normal size.
    e. *Children* require less force, approximately that needed to inflate an ordinary toy balloon.

f. *Infants* are given only short puffs.

C. CLOSED CHEST CARDIAC COMPRESSION (*C* for Circulation)

1. Anatomic Considerations.

Pressure on the sternum compresses the heart and reduces the size of the thoracic cavity. This forces blood out of the ventricles and expels air from lungs. On release, blood flows into the large veins of the chest and into the atria and air enters the lungs.

2. Method.

a. Patient remains in a supine position on a hard surface such as a tray or the floor, if necessary.

b. The heel of the right hand with the heel of the left on top is placed on the lower third of the sternum just above the xiphoid.

c. Firm pressure is applied downward and body weight brought forward to secure sufficient pressure. The sternum should move 4-6 cm. toward the vertebral column in adults. The force is transmitted directly to the heart behind the sternum. *DO NOT* exert pressure on rib cage or epigastrium.

d. Hands should be quickly removed after each application of pressure to allow intrathoracic venous filling and the lungs to expand.

e. Rate of pressure application should be 80 times per minute, slightly faster in children and infants. Also, the force applied must be moderated to fit the elastic properties of the thoracic cage. All that is needed is simple first and middle finger compression in the newborn infant.

f. Observations for the signs of restoration of flow include a full carotid or femoral pulse, constricted pupils, return of skin color, spontaneous ventilation and movements.

g. A systolic blood pressure of 60-80 mm. Hg can be obtained if cardiac compression is correctly performed.

    h.   The ratio of lung inflation (mouth-to-mouth breathing) to cardiac compression should be 1:5 when there is an assistant, and 2:15 (lung to heart) before help arrives.

D. OPEN CHEST RESUSCITATION

1. There are certain situations when emergency thoracotomy and manual cardiac compression is the most effective approach. These include:
   a. Penetrating cardiac injuries, especially with pericardial tamponade.
   b. Flail chest.
   c. Abnormally stiff "emphysematous" thoracic cage.
   d. Air embolism.
   e. If 3-5 minutes of closed massage is ineffective.
2. An emergency anterior thoracotomy is made in the fifth or sixth intercostal space. The ribs are spread with a rib-spreader.
3. The pericardium is incised vertically to *avoid the phrenic nerve.*
4. The entire heart is then grasped and the blood is milked out by applying pressure first to the apex and lastly to the region of the outflow tract. Any cardiac perforations are simultaneously tamponaded with a finger of the other hand until repair can be accomplished.

E. CARDIAC ACTIVATION

1. Definitive therapy begins by alerting the cardiac team, assessing the general condition of the patient, the events surrounding the arrest and continuing the initial resuscitative measures.
2. Sudden cessation of effective cardiac action may be due to either failure of pulse wave formation (*cardiac standstill*) or ineffective pulse wave formation (*ventricular fibrillation*).
3. About 75% of all cardiac arrests in patients are caused by ventricular fibrillation; many of these are

resuscitable. Because of this, electrical defibrillation is recommended early after establishing the
diagnosis by electrocardiograph (chest lead III) or a
cardioscope.

F. VENTRICULAR FIBRILLATION

1. Immediately upon recognition of ventricular tachycardia or fibrillation, a sharp precordial thump with
   the closed fist is delivered. This important first
   maneuver is sometimes effective by depolarizing the
   myocardium and allows for a normal rhythm to develop.
2. If ineffective, *electrical defibrillation* is performed.
   Conductive jelly is applied to the defibrillation pad-
   dles, which are firmly placed on the chest, one over
   the upper sternum and the other to the right of the
   lower sternum (cardiac apex).
3. Only capacitor discharge (DC) defibrillators should
   be used; AC defibrillation is hazardous and may
   cause serious burns.
4. The meter is set at about 400 watt-seconds (joules).
   All attendants are instructed to stand clear of the
   bed or supporting structures. The ECG machine
   must be turned off if it is not internally grounded
   during countershock. *Considerably less voltage* is
   applied to children or to the exposed heart.
5. Secure an electrocardiographic tracing as soon as
   possible and continue specific therapy as indicated
   by the tracing.
6. Give epinephrine or isoproterenol and sodium bicarbonate as described below. These drugs strength-
   en the contractions and permit easier defibrillation.

G. DRUGS (D) (See table)

Start centrally placed intravenous infusion in all cases
(subclavian or jugular veins).

1. *Epinephrine,* dilute (1:10,000), inject 10 ml. I.V. or
   carefully inject 1-2 ml. directly into the ventricle.
   Care must be taken not to tear a coronary vessel.

DRUG THERAPY IN CARDIAC RESUSCITATION

1. Asystole

    a. I.V.* or I.C.+ epinephrine 0.5-1.0 mg. every 3-5 min.
    b. I.V. sodium bicarbonate 44 mEq. every 5-10 min.†
    c. I.V. or I.C. calcium chloride 0.5-1.0 Gm. every 5-10 min.

2. Profound Cardiovascular Collapse

    a. I.V. or I.C. calcium chloride 0.5-1.0 Gm. every 5-10 min.†
    b. I.V. sodium bicarbonate 44 mEq. every 5-10 min.
    c. I.V. or I.C. epinephrine 0.5-1.0 mg. every 3-5 min.†

3. Ventricular Fibrillation

    a. Poor fibrillations
        1) I.V. or I.C. epinephrine 0.5-1.0 mg. every 3-5 min.
        2) I.V. sodium bicarbonate 44 mEq. every 5-10 min.
        3) I.V. lidocaine hydrochloride 50-100 mg., as necessary
    b. Good fibrillations
        1) I.V. lidocaine hydrochloride 50-100 mg., as necessary

---

*Intravenous
+Intracardiac
†See text

2. *Isoproterenol* (Isuprel), dilute (1:50,000), i.e., 0.2 mg. in 10 ml. diluent, I.V., or 0.02 mg. in 10 ml. diluent by intracardiac injection.
3. Continue closed chest compression.
4. Sodium bicarbonate, 44.6 mEq. (50 ml. of 7.5% concentration) I.V., initially (smaller doses in children). Repeat $NaHCO_3$ every 5-10 minutes if arrest persists (monitor with blood pH data).
5. Repeat epinephrine and/or isoproterenol injections every 5 minutes.
6. Calcium chloride, 10% solution. A short time after the first isoproterenol injection, inject 5-10 ml. Calcium helps to restore cellular membrane potential and augments isoproterenol effectiveness.

7. Lidocaine hydrochloride (Xylocaine) 50-100 mg. in 2.5 or 5 ml. of a 2% solution should be given rapidly. An infusion of 500 mg. in 500 ml. of 5% glucose in water can help maintain rhythm.

III. SELECTION OF PATIENTS

Keen judgment must be used on wards and in the Emergency Service in the selection of patients for whom resuscitative efforts are to be expended. In my opinion, resuscitation should not be instituted on all patients. When, in the judgment of the physician there is little hope for the establishment of sustained spontaneous cardiac and respiratory action and when there is little hope for a successful outcome, it is my opinion resuscitation measures of this type should not be instituted or pursued. Thus, I do not believe patients with advanced cardiovascular or renal disease or inoperable carcinoma should be treated.

Objective:

Restoration of oxygen delivery to body tissues by simple means is recommended for patients in whom cardiac arrest has been precipitated by accidental means or by certain natural disease processes. The technique presented obviates the need for thoracotomy and specialized equipment in most circumstances.

CHAPTER 2

Emergency Care of Acute Myocardial Infarction

EDWARD B. J. WINSLOW, M.D., F.R.C.P. (C)

I. DEFINITION

A. *Acute Myocardial Infarction* (AMI) occurs when there is myocardial necrosis. This is usually associated with coronary atherosclerosis and frequently with thrombosis of one or more of the coronary arteries.

1. *Clinical definition:* A history of chest pain in patients who might logically be expected to develop this problem because of age and/or the presence of coronary risk factors.
2. The patient with AMI is very fragile and stands a good chance of dying of ventricular arrhythmias within the first few hours of the onset of the infarction (1, 2).
3. The hospital Emergency Service may be the first place that he will come for care.
4. It is very often the initial care that determines whether he lives or dies.
5. It is *mandatory* that patients who might have AMI be evaluated and treated promptly and correctly.

II. DIAGNOSIS

A. The diagnosis of AMI usually is made from the history and confirmed with laboratory studies.

1. The *history* may be very suggestive, with a "crushing" substernal chest pain, radiation down the arm associated with diaphoresis and shortness of breath and anxiety.

2. The history may not be so definite and, even in the very intelligent patient, the diagnosis of AMI may be elusive.
3. *Any* middle-aged patient, or man in the fourth decade or older, who presents with chest pains, however vague, should be treated as a patient with AMI until the diagnosis can be confirmed or excluded.
4. It is the efficiency with which the first few minutes of contact with the hospital is conducted that often will determine the eventual outcome.

B. MONITORING

1. The patient with a suspect AMI should *first* be monitored with an electrocardiogram before *anything* else is done.
2. He should be attached to a cardiac monitor so that during his *whole stay* in the Emergency Service his cardiac rhythm can be observed while a history is taken and administrative details are completed.
3. The most important thing during this phase of the patient's course is his cardiac rhythm.
4. One should choose an ECG lead that will give the most information.
5. This lead is usually lead V_1 and is often difficult to set up on a set of monitor leads.
6. The *recommended* monitor lead is a modified lead CL_1, as illustrated in Figure 2-1 (3).
7. If a monitor is not available, then the patient should be attached to a standard ECG machine and a 12-lead ECG taken. The machine should *not* be disconnected until a decision has been made about the patient's diagnosis and disposition.

C. The *diagnosis* of AMI should be considered seriously in *all* patients with chest pain, especially if this chest pain was preceded by any effort-induced pain relieved by rest or nitroglycerin (angina pectoris).
1. If this pain began within the few weeks preceding the present episode or if previously existing angina has increased in frequency or severity, then the diagnosis of AMI should be very strongly suspected.

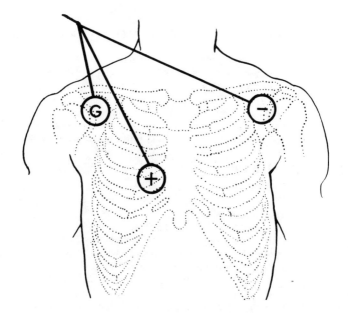

PREVENTION

Fig. 2-1.—Modified CL₁ lead. (*G*), ground lead; (-), negative lead, usually labeled RA; (+), positive lead, usually labeled LA, or foot.

2. The *pain* of AMI is usually of longer duration and greater intensity than the patient's existing angina and is frequently associated with other symptoms such as dyspnea, diaphoresis, nausea, vomiting or the urge to defecate. However, AMI can present with many other varied symptoms, especially epigastric, back, shoulder or arm pain.
3. AMI may be the cause for worsening of *congestive heart failure* or the onset of *acute pulmonary edema.*
4. It may likewise present as a syncopal episode or a stroke.

5. The ECG is helpful only if it shows changes that are compatible with the diagnosis of AMI.
6. A patient with a *strongly suggestive history* but a *normal ECG should never* be dismissed as normal until a very careful examination has shown another reason for his pain and until he is stable.
7. It has been shown repeatedly that many patients who die from AMI and its associated arrhythmias had seen a physician within the preceding few days.

III. PHYSICAL EXAMINATION

A. The examination of a patient with acute myocardial infarction may be very unrevealing.
   1. An atrial gallop is usually heard over the left ventricular apex or in the suprasternal notch. The frequency with which this sound is heard is directly proportional to the experience of the examiner and the diligence with which the sound is sought.
   2. Often this is the *only* abnormal physical finding in the patient with AMI other than apprehension and diaphoresis.
   3. Findings such as pulmonary edema or shock are often present and may be more prominent than those signs peculiar to AMI.

IV. ELECTROCARDIOGRAM

The ECG may show Q wave or ST-T wave changes that are easily recognized. However, it often may be normal or show only nonspecific ST-T wave changes.

V. TREATMENT

A. Treatment of patients with AMI is directed at:
   1. Relief of pain.
   2. Relief of apprehension.
   3. Treatment of arrhythmias.
   4. Treatment of other complications such as shock or congestive heart failure.

B. *Sudden arrhythmias* are frequent in patients with AMI.
   1. Treatment of these arrhythmias must be rapid, and
      because the confirmation of the diagnosis may rest
      on tests of *muscle enzymes*, an intravenous line
      should be established, preferably with a plastic
      cannula.
   2. All medications should be given intravenously for
      two reasons:
      a. I.M. injections interfere with other tests.
      b. I.M. injections are often erratically absorbed be-
         cause of vasoconstriction.
   3. Oxygen is given by a well-fitting mask or by nasal
      catheter at 8-10 liters per minute.
   4. After the I.V. line has been established, *pain* should
      be relieved (4). There are several drugs that are ef-
      fective in relieving the pain of AMI:
      a. Morphine, 5-10 mg. given I.V. in 1-mg. aliquots,
         is the oldest agent and the drug of choice. Al-
         though it can cause orthostatic hypotension,
         this should be no problem because the patient
         should be supine for monitoring.
         1) If hypotension occurs, elevating the feet may
            be effective.
      b. Pentazocine (Talwin), 30-60 mg. I.V., is also ef-
         fective and is claimed to have little cardiodepres-
         sor effect.
      c. Meperidine (Demerol) hydrochloride, 25-50 mg.
         I.V., may also be useful.

C. Treatment of *arrhythmias* is aimed at *preventing* the development of *ventricular tachycardia* or *ventricular
   fibrillation*.
   1. These arrhythmias are often difficult to treat.
   2. There are many theories about which rhythms are
      dangerous.
   3. The most commonly accepted signs of impending
      ventricular fibrillation are ventricular arrhythmias,
      which may occur:
      a. Early in the cycle, with interruption of the T
         wave (R on T phenomenon).

      b. In salvos of two or more.

      c. In multiform configuration.

      d. With sustained contraction and at a frequency of greater than 5 per minute.

4. The *treatment* for these arrhythmias is lidocaine (Xylocaine) hydrochloride, 50-100 mg., by I.V. bolus followed by a constant infusion by drip at 1-3 mg. per minute.

      a. *Ventricular tachycardia* requires individualized treatment.

          1) If the patient is still awake and has palpable pulses, conversion to sinus rhythm may be accomplished with lidocaine (100 mg. I.V.).

          2) If the patient becomes unconscious or is losing consciousness, he should be cardioverted *immediately* using 400 watt-seconds D.C. countershock.

          3) The paddles are placed on the anterior chest, one at the third right intercostal space and the other over the cardiac apex.

          4) The ECG machine should be disconnected prior to administering the shock so that the machine does not get blown out.

      b. *Ventricular fibrillation*

          1) Cardiopulmonary resuscitation must be instituted immediately (see Chap. 1) *by administering countershock.*

          2) If sinus rhythm is restored, lidocaine should be given I.V., 2 mg. per minute.

      c. *Bradyarrhythmias*

          1) These may be *sinus bradycardias* or *atrioventricular blocks.*

          2) Treatment depends upon both the type of bradyarrhythmia and the patient's response to the treatment.

             a) When sinus bradycardia is associated with premature ventricular contractions, they may be abolished simply by speeding up the cardiac rate with atropine (0.4-1.0 mg. I.V.).

b) When atrioventricular block has occurred
with inferior wall AMI and narrow QRS
complexes (less than 0.10 second), the
ventricular response can often be speed-
ed up with *isoproterenol* infusions at a
rate of 2-3 μg. per minute.

c) A-V block with wide QRS complexes
is best managed with transvenous pac-
ing, but, while waiting to get the pacemaker in, *isoproterenol* should be
given.

d) Because of the fragility of the patient
and the time involved in transporting
him to the cardiac care unit (C.C.U.) he
should be *stable*, with *arrhythmias
treated before* he is moved, and he
should be accompanied to the C.C.U. by
a physician or a nurse.

VI. SHOCK

A. Shock occurring in the presence of AMI is an ominous
sign and must be treated rapidly. In general, shock in
the *absence* of arrhythmias signifies:
1. A very extensive infarction.
2. Hypovolemia caused by:
   a. Over-vigorous use of diuretics.
   b. The patient's apprehension, leading to decreased
   oral intake of fluids.

B. The *diagnosis* of shock is made from:
1. Signs of poor tissue perfusion.
2. Cool, clammy skin.
3. Peripheral cyanosis.
4. Obtunded mentation.
5. Tachycardia.
6. Oliguria (urine flow of less than 0.5 ml. per minute).
7. Hypotension.
8. A significant drop from a previously high blood
pressure.

C. Treatment is directed at improving tissue perfusion and oxygenation.
1. If the blood pressure is less than 80 mm. Hg systolic, administer a vasopressor. We prefer norepinephrine (Levarterenol [Levophed] bitartrate). *Dose: one ampul* (4 ml.), mixed in 250 ml. of 5% dextrose in water (D5W) through a microdrip.
2. This should be given through a *well* inserted, *freely* running catheter.
3. Extravasation will damage all tissues and may cause a skin slough.
4. If this should occur, immediately infiltrate freely with *phentolamine (Regitine), 5-10 mg.* in *10-15 ml. of saline, 0.9%.*
5. When the blood pressure is between 80-100 mm. Hg systolic, a *volume challenge* should be given.
6. In the Emergency Service this procedure can be monitored by:
   a. Pulse rate.
   b. Blood pressure.
   c. Central venous pressure (CVP).
   d. Urine flow.
   e. Clinical observation of the patient's tissue perfusion.
7. After baseline measurements are taken and recorded, 100 ml. of fluid (D5W: lactated Ringer's solution, 0.9% sodium chloride and low mol. wt. dextran) is given over a 5-10-minute period and a repeat set of measurements is taken.
8. Monitoring is repeated until:
   a. The patient recovers.
   b. Congestive heart failure, rales in the chest, etc., occur.
   c. The CVP increases 2 (or more) ml. H_2O after a 100 ml. volume challenge.

SAMPLE FLOW CHART

Time	BP	P	CVP	Urine Flow	Skin	Mental Status	Medication: Norepinephrine	Fluid Volume
9:00	80/60	110	5	0 ml.	Cool, clammy	Confused	2 ml./min.	None
9:10	85/60	110	5	0 ml.	Cool, clammy	Confused	2 ml./min.	D5W, 100 ml.
9:20	85/60	115	5	10 ml.	Cool, dry	Confused	2 ml./min.	D5W, 100 ml.
9:30	85/60	120	8*	5 ml.	Cool, dry	Confused	2 ml./min.	D5W, 100 ml.

*The volume challenge is stopped because of the CVP rise of 3 cm. During a volume challenge there should be *no change in drug administration*.

REFERENCES

1. Grace, W. J.: The mobile coronary care unit and the intermediate coronary care unit in the total systems approach to coronary care, Chest 58:363, 1970.
2. Yu, P. N., et al.: Resources for the optimal care of patients with acute myocardial infarction, Circulation 43:A-171, 1971.
3. Marriott, H. J. L.: Prevention and Treatment of Cardiac Arrhythmias Associated with Myocardial Infarction; Coronary Heart Disease, in Brest, A. N. (ed.): *Coronary Heart Disease* (Philadelphia: F. A. Davis Co., 1969).
4. Todres, D.: The role of morphine in acute myocardial infarction, Am. Heart J. 81:566, 1971.
5. Lown, B., et al.: The coronary care unit. New perspectives and didirections, J.A.M.A. 199:156, 1967.

As soon as the patient is stable, he should be transferred to the C.C.U., where he can be observed closely and treated vigorously (5).

CHAPTER 3

Principles in Treatment of Wounds

JOHN H. SCHNEEWIND, M.D.

I. INCISED WOUNDS

See Chapters 4 and 5.

A. Incised wounds may be closed by primary suture if:
1. They are seen within 6-8 hours after injury.
2. They are *not* of the puncture type—that is, one with a small entrance and narrow, deep tract.
3. They have been protected by a clean, adequate dressing.

B. Patients with badly contaminated wounds that require extensive debridement must be *admitted* and treated in the hospital operating rooms.

C. Tetanus prophylaxis must be considered (Chap. 7).

D. **Technique**
1. Do a preliminary examination in a clean area.
2. Wear a cap and mask and have available the sterile instruments and bandages necessary to protect the wound against further contamination.
3. Test for injury to underlying structures (bone, muscles, tendons, nerves and vessels) by inspecting wound and examining areas proximal and distal.
   a. *Do not probe* wound.
   b. If a vital structure is damaged, obtain surgical consultation.
4. Scrub hands and arms in accordance with "Scrub Techniques" (see below).
5. Prepare skin (see below).

41

6. Explore wound and remove foreign material.
    a. Extensive debridement must be carried out in wounds badly contaminated with dirt and foreign bodies.
    b. Clean wounds may require little or no debridement, although all devitalized tissue must be excised.
    c. After debridement, every recess should be thoroughly lavaged with warm, sterile saline solution.
7. Obtain hemostasis by carefully clamping and ligating bleeding vessels.
8. Repair wound by sutures in such a way that *no dead space remains* (see Chap. 4).

E. For management of contused, stellate and slicing (beveled) wounds and the appropriate suture materials and techniques see Chapter 4, "Management of Facial Injuries."

II. PUNCTURE WOUNDS

A. The wound of entrance is small with a narrow, deep tract.
    1. This is a tetanus-prone injury.
    2. It may be preferable to convert these into open wounds in order to irrigate and debride them thoroughly.
    3. The wound may then possibly be safe to suture primarily.
    4. Always test for injury to bone, muscles, tendons, nerves and large vessels by examining areas proximal and distal to the wounds. *Do not probe wound.*

B. **Technique**

    1. Clean surrounding skin with soap and water for 10 minutes. Remove soap with warm, sterile saline. *Do not attempt* to wash out or irrigate wound itself.

2. Wound edges must be kept open so that if pus forms, it can drain to the outside.
   a. If wound edges appear likely to seal over, a small ellipse of skin may be removed.
   b. A small wick of moist gauze may be put just below the skin edges.
   c. *Do not* use iodoform.

3. Cover with sterile dressings and immobilize part.

C. Specimens should be taken for a gram-stain, culture and sensitivity studies.

D. Antibiotics often are indicated (see Part I, "Antibiotics in the Emergency Service," and Chap. 5).

III. ANIMAL BITE WOUNDS

A. Clean skin surrounding wound with soap and water for 10 minutes. Remove soap with warm, sterile saline water.

B. Do not irrigate the wound if it is a puncture type.

C. If the wound is wide open, it should be irrigated and debrided thoroughly.

D. Keep wound open with sterile, wet dressings. *Primary suture rarely should be done,* except in extensive injuries, notably to the face.

   Note: For *human bite wounds,* the treatment is similar except that *such wounds never are primarily sutured.*

IV. SCRUB TECHNIQUES

A. Wash hands and arms thoroughly to 2 inches above elbows with plain soap and then rinse. Repeat two additional times.

B. Clean nails with file.

C. Scrub hands and arms thoroughly, using brush and soap (or antiseptic) for 10 minutes.

D. Dry hands and forearms with sterile towel.

E. If patient has not been prepared, put on sterile gloves and prepare patient in accordance with techniques for "Preparation of Patient" (see below). Do not contaminate bare arms.

F. After preparing patient, rescrub for 3 minutes. Again dry hands.

G. Don sterile gown, being careful not to contaminate it by brushing against nonsterile objects.

H. Put on sterile gloves.

I. Drape the patient.

V. PREPARATION OF PATIENT

A. A cap and mask should be worn by the nurse and patient.

B. Open a sterile preparation pack. Scrub hands and arms as described above.

C. If the injured part is an extremity, the patient is asked to elevate it and sterile towels are placed beneath it. Wash entire circumference well above and below the wound.

D. Wash *around* wound thoroughly for 10 minutes with soap and sterile water.

E. Irrigate the wound thoroughly with physiologic saline solution.

F. Apply antiseptic solution to skin around wound—*not in* the wound.

G. *Remove all wet or contaminated drapes.*

H. Use fresh sterile towels or sheets to redrape.

I. Draping for facial lacerations is illustrated in Chapter 4. *Note:* Scalp wounds should have hair removed for 4 inches from wounds on all sides. This applies to most other wounds.

J. *Do not shave eyebrows.*
    1. They are an invaluable landmark for precise reap-
        proximation.
    2. If shaved, they often grow back abnormally.
    3. They may be clipped.

VI. RECORDS

It is mandatory that all of the following information be
recorded.

A. Date and time of injury.
B. Cause and location of injury.
C. Site, location, depth and size of wound.
D. Associated nerve, vascular, muscle, tendon or bone in-
    jury if present. (A note should be made if these struc-
    tures are intact.)
E. Type of anesthesia.
F. Number of sutures.
G. Presence or absence of other injuries.
H. Impression.
I. Disposition.
J. All instructions must be given to the patient *in writing*
    and a copy made part of the Emergency Service Record.
    These *include* a return appointment or referral to the
    patient's own physician.

CHAPTER 4

Management of Facial Injuries

PAUL W. GREELEY, M.D., A. GILMAN MIDDLE-
TON, M.D., *and* JOHN W. CURTIN, M.D.

I. INTRODUCTION

A. In treating facial injuries, the entire patient must be evaluated to establish proper priority of management when
there are multiple body wounds.

B. Definitive repair of facial wounds can be delayed several
hours if necessary. Reduction of fractures may even be
postponed for several days until the soft-tissue swelling
has subsided, at which time the patient's general condition will permit surgical correction.

C. Adequate anesthesia must always be provided (see Chap.
5 and 6).
   1. Local infiltration with 1% lidocaine is ideal for
      wound closures in cooperative adults.
   2. In dealing with extensive wounds or with wounds in
      children, endotracheal general anesthesia is prefer-
      able.

D. All wounds must be treated in a well-equipped operating
room, with the necessary medical and nursing personnel,
if poor results are to be avoided.

E. If a complicated or extensive problem is presented, the
patient should be transferred at once to the main operating suite.

F. For closure of lacerated wounds, fine, delicate instruments are needed.
   1. Surgical trauma must be minimized.

2. Small bleeding points are ligated with fine sutures.
3. Skin edges are approximated with fine interrupted sutures of 5-0 or 6-0 monofilament nylon swedged into fine curved cutting needles.
4. Interrupted sutures are placed approximately 1/8 inch apart in order to obtain accurate coaptation of the skin edges. Needles must enter and exit *perpendicular* to the skin!

II. GENERAL WOUND CARE

A. General surgical principles apply to facial injuries as to those of other regions, including the prevention of infection and tetanus prophylaxis.

B. However, primary repair of certain facial wounds may be done many hours after initial emergency cure has been administered.

C. The face must be prepared with sterile cotton, soap and water, followed by aqueous Zephiran; with copious lavage of the wounds with sterile saline solution.

D. Antiseptics containing alcohol, iodine, etc., should not be used because they serve only to cauterize the healthy wound borders and incite inflammatory reaction in the wound.

E. Hair should be shaved around the wound, but *not the eyebrows* (since they are a valuable guide for realignment of tissues).

F. Draping with towels rather than "peephole" sheets generally helps maintain a clean, unobstructed field (Fig. 4-1).

G. Foreign debris and devitalized tissue are removed; however, debridement is limited to obviously necrotic tissue, particularly in wounds near the eyelid, nose, etc., where a few millimeters may be a disastrous loss.

H. Thorough hemostasis must be achieved with 4-0 plain catgut ligatures followed by meticulous wound closure.

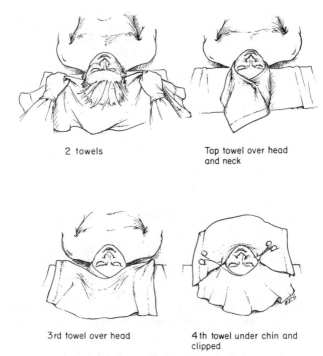

2 towels

Top towel over head
and neck

3rd towel over head

4th towel under chin and
clipped

Fig. 4-1.—Draping for facial injuries.

I. Pressure dressings generally are applied to absorb wound drainage, control hematomas and minimize postoperative edema.

III. THE UNTIDY WOUND

A. The grossly contused, "untidy," irregular laceration is probably best handled by:
1. Wound excision to obtain precise borders.
2. Undermining of the wound edges and careful suturing (i.e., with 5-0 or 6-0 nylon sutures) (Fig. 4-2).

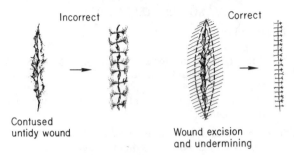

Incorrect   Correct

Contused
untidy wound

Wound excision
and undermining

Fig. 4-2.–Skin laceration.

B. This cannot be done where a feature such as the eyelid
    is involved, for distortion would result.

IV. MUSCLE REPAIR

A. Where muscle is severed, a two-layered closure is impor-
    tant. If it is not employed, the muscle will retract, with
    hematoma filling the gap, and the resultant scar will con-
    tract and become a depressed skin scar (Fig. 4-3).

B. Muscle layers may be repaired with 3-0 or 4-0 chromic
    catgut or nylon.

Fig. 4-3.–Muscle injury.

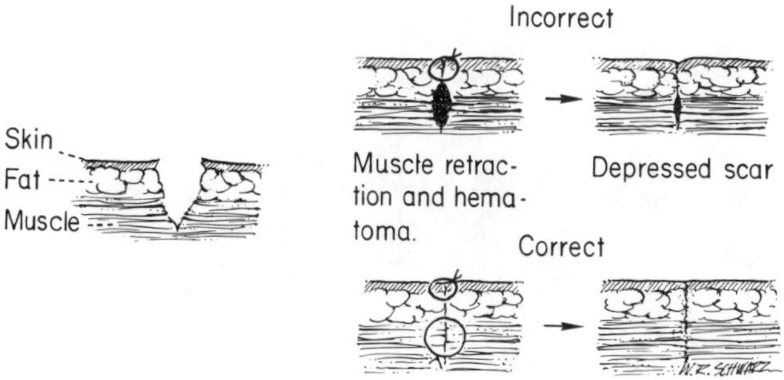

Incorrect

Skin
Fat
Muscle

Muscle retrac-
tion and hema-
toma.

Depressed scar

Correct

V. SUTURE TECHNIQUE

A. Suggested suture materials:
1. Skin—5-0 or 6-0 nylon.
2. Subcutaneous sutures and hemostatic ligatures—4-0 or 5-0 plain catgut or nylon.
3. Muscle—3-0 or 4-0 nylon.
4. Mucosa—4-0 nylon. (If infection is likely, use chromic catgut.)

B. The final result is related directly to the care taken by the Emergency Service surgeon in wound repair.

Fig. 4-4.—Suture tension.

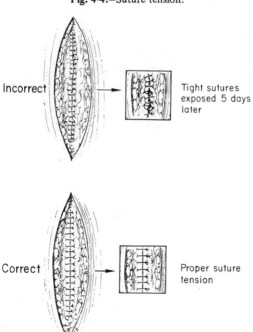

Incorrect → Tight sutures exposed 5 days later

Correct → Proper suture tension

1. Fine instruments and meticulous care in handling the tissues are basic requirements.
2. Sutures must just approximate tissues (Fig. 4-4).
3. Tight sutures cause tissue necrosis and gross delay in wound healing, and produce "railroad ties" across an otherwise satisfactory scar (Fig. 4-5).
4. Simple sutures taking in sufficient and equal amounts of subcutaneous and dermal tissue will usually give good wound approximation, while small horizontal mattress sutures spaced as necessary may help to evert the edges.
5. Improper repair results in rolled edges, leaving unsightly scars. Wide mattress sutures are never needed in facial repair.

C. Poor scars result from:
   1. Suture material that is too heavy.
   2. Inclusion of too much tissue in the suture.
   3. Sutures that are too tight.
   4. Delayed removal of sutures.

Fig. 4-5.—Suture technique.

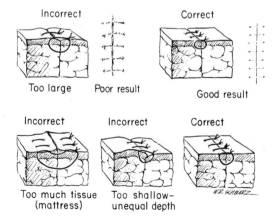

Incorrect

Too large   Poor result

Correct

Good result

Incorrect

Too much tissue (mattress)

Incorrect

Too shallow— unequal depth

Correct

D. Sutures may be removed *from the face* between the third and fifth days. If in doubt about the integrity of the wound, support it with sterile adhesive butterfly or collodion strips.

VI. TYPES OF WOUNDS

A. *Stellate or "V"-shaped lacerations* may present an ischemic skin flap.
    1. Care should be taken to avoid strangulation of the tip by sutures.
    2. A "corner suture" picking up only dermis in the tip may help in alignment (Fig. 4-6).

B. *Slicing wounds* with beveled edges will often heal with contraction along the oblique tract of fibrous tissue, producing a rolled or pouting wound margin (Fig. 4-7).
    1. This will be even more apparent in the "trap door" wound, where the circular scar also contracts, causing further pouting in the wound margin.
    2. Trimming the border to vertical or stepped edges will result in a better scar.

Fig. 4-6.—Stellate lacerations.

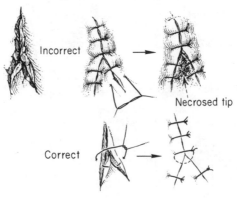

Incorrect

Necrosed tip

Correct

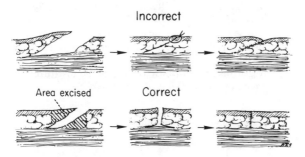

Incorrect

Area excised   Correct

Suture Materials :

Muscle	4-0 Chromic catgut
Subcuti-cular ligatures	4-0 Plain catgut
Skin	5-0 or 6-0 Nylon (silk)

Fig. 4-7.—Slicing wound.

C. Where a flap of tissue is avulsed on a small pedicle, the arterial supply may exceed the venous and lymphatic drainage, resulting in venous congestion and necrosis. Severing the attachment and treating the tissue as a free graft (after defatting) will assure a more satisfactory "take."

VII. BITES

See Chapter 5, "Injuries and Infections of the Hand."

A. Animal bites with puncture wounds should not be irrigated or closed.

B. If extensive tissue tearing is present, particularly on the face, primary repair after prolonged cleansing and debridement is indicated.

C. Human bites are generally seen late and are likely to be severely infected.
   1. Those involving the face (usually the nose or ear), however, may benefit from primary repair if seen immediately after the injury.
   2. Vigorous antibiotic therapy must be instituted immediately (see Part 1, 4, and Chap. 5).

Fig. 4-8.—Through and through lip laceration.

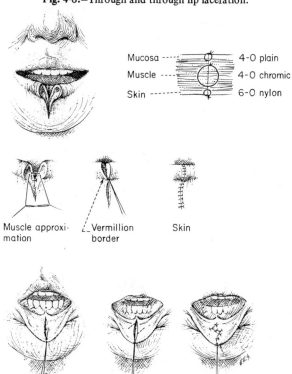

Mucosa ---- 4-0 plain
Muscle ---- 4-0 chromic
Skin ------ 6-0 nylon

Muscle approximation

Vermillion border

Skin

Repair of mucosa with Z-plasty

VIII. TONGUE AND ORAL MUCOSA

A. Common lacerations of the tongue and lips produced by the teeth generally heal satisfactorily without sutures.

B. Through-and-through lacerations of the cheek or lip require:
1. Careful muscle approximation.
2. Closure of the oral mucosa.
3. Precise skin approximation.

C. Precise alignment of the vermilion border of the lip is *most* important (Fig. 4-8).

D. Postoperatively, a liquid diet and mouthwash will keep most wounds clean.

E. Frequent swabbing of the skin wound with cotton applicators saturated with 3% hydrogen peroxide will prevent crusting and subsequent purulent collections.

IX. EYELID LACERATIONS

A. Eyelid lacerations must be repaired in the main operating suite, where proper instruments, suture material and personnel are available. A simple straight-line repair may result in a surgical coloboma of the lid from scar contracture (Fig. 4-9).

B. Always remember that time of removal of skin sutures will vary with their location and the degree of wound tension.
1. Thin skin, such as that of the eyelids, heals quickly; hence, sutures can be removed in 2-3 days.
2. Thicker skin of the face and in those areas subject to muscle pull heals more slowly.
3. However, all sutures must be taken out before any inflammation can develop around them.
4. If stitches are left in place, such minor points of inflammation about them invariably lead to local suppuration—the cause of stitch-hole scars.

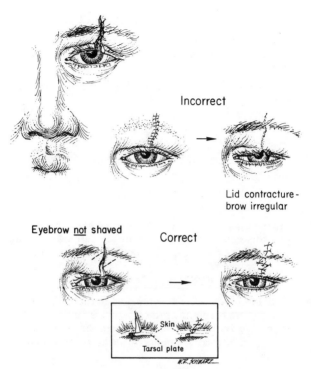

Fig. 4-9.—Eyelid lacerations.

X. INGROUND FOREIGN MATERIAL

A. After cleansing, the wound is inspected carefully with a magnifying lens or loupe. Strict attention is paid to the presence of any foreign material.
   1. This must be removed at once, because such foreign material becomes fixed rapidly into the tissue edges of lacerations or into abrasions.
   2. Failure to remove it will leave permanent pigmentation in the skin, commonly referred to as "accidental tattoo."

B. If the foreign material is grease or paint, ether may dissolve it.

C. If it is street dirt or gunpowder, the wound should be scrubbed vigorously with a stiff brush.
   1. If the material is deep or difficult to dislodge, the use of a motor-driven wire brush may be helpful.

D. In case the discoloration is limited to the wound edges only, it may be better to debride these areas with a sharp straight-edge scalpel.

E. After the abraded wound has been treated, it is dressed by covering with sterile fine nylon silk and a gauze dressing, applied under moderate pressure.

XI. AVULSIONS

A. If a large segment of skin has been avulsed, it should always be looked for at the scene of the accident.
   1. It may be used, but this skin has been badly mutilated and a graft may be much safer.
   2. It can be prepared using the same procedure employed to cleanse the wound.
   3. Any underlying fat is trimmed and the skin reapplied to its original bed in the form of a free full-thickness skin graft.

B. Skin flaps that have been partially avulsed are always precarious in their behavior.
   1. Invariably they have a better arterial supply than a venous return.
   2. The lack of good venous supply predisposes to venous congestion and moist gangrene.
   3. Flaps of this type frequently can be saved by *deliberately dividing* the remaining pedicle, removing the underlying attached subcutaneous fat, and then reapplying the skin as a free full-thickness graft.

C. Avulsions of large organs, such as an entire nose or ear, are catastrophes. Successful anastomosis is unlikely because of their large mass.

1. In the case of an avulsed ear, one should remove the overlying skin and salvage the underlying auricular cartilage.
2. These tissues may be buried temporarily in a subcutaneous pocket in the anterior abdominal wall.
3. Later, they can be utilized as ideal structural support in constructing a new ear.

X. DEEP WOUNDS

A. A careful inspection must be made of all deep lacerations.
   1. Divided muscles are reapproximated with interrupted sutures.
   2. The divided ends of Stensen's duct or the facial nerve must be identified and anastomosed with a few interrupted sutures of 6-0 silk in the main operating suite.

B. A special problem is presented by extensive facial wounds which open into the oral cavity.
   1. It is necessary to approximate these wounds in layers in meticulous fashion to restore facial symmetry.
   2. The mucous membrane is included in the reapproximation.
   3. The muscles, subcutaneous tissues and skin are closed in layers.
   4. Should a lacrimal duct be divided, it must be sutured at once, using a small internal polyethylene tube to splint the severed duct ends.
   5. Likewise, divided internal or external palpebral ligaments should be repaired primarily.
   6. This type of injury is repaired in the main operating suite.

XI. INFECTED WOUNDS

A. In general, infected facial wounds should be treated with continual warm, moist dressings with frequent changes.

B. Specimens are taken for a gram stain, culture and sensitivity studies.

C. Antibiotics are prescribed (see Part I, "Antibiotics in the Emergency Service," and Chap. 5).

XII. FACIAL BONE FRACTURES

Clinical diagnosis of facial bone fractures can be made with a high degree of accuracy.

A. An ecchymotic orbit is suggestive of a *Malar Bone Fracture* (Fig. 4-10). The possibility is made quite certain by:
   1. Palpable irregularities and depression of the orbital floor.

Fig. 4-10.—Depressed fracture of right malar bone.

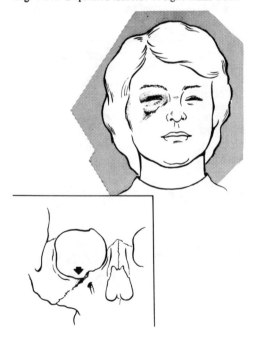

   2. Flattening and depression of the malar eminence.
   3. Subjective complaints of diplopia and numbness
      along the distribution of the infraorbital nerve.

B. A *Blow-out Fracture* of the orbital floor may occur
   along with other fractures of the malar bone or as a separate entity.
   1. Noting that the eyeball is resting at a lower level
      facilitates recognition of this fracture.
   2. Accurate diagnosis is confirmed by adequate x-ray
      studies.

C. A visible or palpable depression over the *Zygomatic
   Arch* suggests a depressed fracture (Fig. 4-11) in this

Fig. 4-11.—Depressed fracture of zygomatic arch.

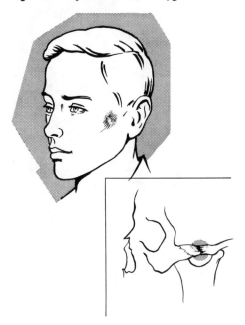

area. Depression of the bony fragments against the underlying coronoid process and temporalis muscle may make opening of the mouth difficult or impossible.

D. Tenderness along the mandible in one or more areas, along with irregularity of the lower teeth, suggests a *Mandibular Fracture.*

E. The *Maxilla,* if badly injured, may be movable and even be dropping into the mouth.

F. *Nasal Fractures* are usually depressed or lateral, depending on whether the blow was applied from in front or from one side. Inspection of the nostrils may reveal a *Septal Cartilage Dislocation* into either nasal airway.

G. For obvious surgical and medicolegal reasons, all of the foregoing clinical findings must be verified by special x-ray studies.

H. **Treatment**
   1. The reduction and the immobilization of facial bone fractures are not necessarily surgical emergencies.
   2. Because extensive soft-tissue swelling usually accompanies facial bone fractures, it may be advantageous to wait a few days for this edema to subside.
   3. Surgery will be easier and maintenance of position will become less difficult.
   4. It may be the opinion of the attending surgeon that certain simple mandibular fractures can be treated by interdental wiring or elastic traction.
      a. In such cases, consultation with a dentist trained in this field will be helpful.
      b. All complicated fractures of the mandible and maxilla require open reduction.
      c. Nasal fractures and septal dislocations customarily are treated by closed reduction. It is advisable to manipulate septal cartilage dislocations as early as possible.
         1) Hematoma formation around the cartilage is frequent. The hematoma provides an excellent culture medium that in turn leads to a septal abscess.

2) This is likely to progress to septic chondritis and loss of the septal cartilage, leaving the patient with a saddle deformity of the nose.

5. For all complicated fractures of the mandible, maxilla, central third of the face and malar-zygomatic bones, open reduction invariably is indicated.

    a. For these cases, it is wise to obtain consultation with a plastic surgeon.

    b. Definitive treatment should be delayed several days until much of the facial edema has subsided.

    c. Two or three weeks' delay is not unusual in cases of severe and extensive injuries.

    d. They are never surgical emergencies, provided an *adequate airway* has been established.

XIII. ANESTHESIA FOR FACIAL BONE FRACTURES

Anesthesia is very important.

A. Local anesthesia works very well with nasal fractures and septal dislocations, except in small children.

    1. The nostrils are packed with cotton pledgets soaked in equal parts of 1:1000 adrenalin and a 10% solution of cocaine or Pontocaine.

    2. The soft tissues are infiltrated with 1% Xylocaine or Novocain, to which 5 or 10 drops of adrenalin are added for each *ounce* of anesthetic agent.

B. For the treatment of the more complicated fractures that necessitate open reduction, endotracheal general anesthesia is mandatory.

    1. It is almost impossible to reduce and wire many mandibular fractures without general anesthesia because of the ever-present associated severe muscle spasms.

CHAPTER 5

Injuries and Infections of the Hand

JOHN H. SCHNEEWIND, M.D.

I. GENERAL PRINCIPLES

A. Evaluation of the patient as a whole must precede diagnosis and treatment of the specific hand injury.
    1. Inquiry must be made whether the patient has a chronic systemic disease such as:
        a. Diabetes mellitus.
        b. Circulatory insufficiency, general or in the hands.
        c. General chronic systemic disease or neoplasm.
    2. It should also be learned whether the patient is receiving steroid therapy and the status of tetanus immunization.
    3. Treatment priorities must be established for the patient with multiple injuries. Life-threatening conditions must be dealt with at once.

B. An accurate history of the specific hand injury must be obtained. Important considerations are:
    1. Time elapsed since injury.
    2. How and where sustained.
    3. Occupation of the patient (injuries sustained by butchers or meat handlers are very susceptible to infection).

C. **TYPES OF INJURY**
    1. Laceration (See Chap. 4, "Management of Facial Injuries").
        a. Tidy (a clean laceration caused by a knife, broken bottle, etc.).

      b. Untidy (avulsed or irregular lacerations with or
         without a crush component).
      c. With possible involvement of tendons, nerves,
         vessels and bone.
  2. Severe crushing of the entire hand.
  3. Multiple fractures—open or closed.
  4. Burns.
  5. Traumatic amputations.

II. FUNCTIONAL ANATOMY OF THE HAND

Accurate diagnosis in injuries and infections makes precise
knowledge of the anatomy mandatory.

Fig. 5-1.—Volar aspect of wrist.

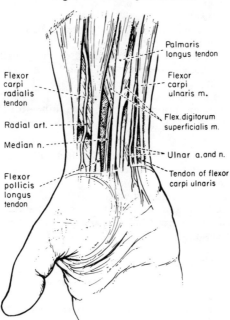

Palmaris
longus tendon

Flexor
carpi
radialis
tendon

Flexor
carpi
ulnaris m.

Radial art.

Flex. digitorum
superficialis m.

Median n.

Ulnar a. and n.

Flexor
pollicis
longus
tendon

Tendon of flexor
carpi ulnaris

A. X-ray films of the bones of the wrist and hand in both adults and children are required. Views of *both* hands and wrist are useful, especially in children.

B. **VOLAR SURFACE OF THE WRIST** (Fig. 5-1)

1. The volar surface of the wrist is divided into radial and ulnar portions by the centrally placed flexor carpi radialis and palmaris longus tendons (approximately 15% of patients do not have a palmaris longus tendon and muscle in one forearm, 7% have none in either forearm).

2. The ulnar border of the wrist is bounded by the flexor carpi ulnaris. Directly beneath it lie the ulnar artery and nerve.

3. Between the radial and ulnar wrist flexors lie *all* of the superficialis and profundus flexor tendons to the fingers. This group does *not* include the flexor pollicis longus.

4. *Radial* to the flexor carpi radialis lie the flexor pollicis longus and the deeper structures of the wrist.

C. **PALM OF HAND**

1. **Superficial Structures** (Fig. 5-2).

    The median and ulnar nerves, superficial volar arch, the superficialis and profundus flexor tendons to the digits and their insertions are shown.

2. **Deep Structures.**

    a. The transverse carpal ligament forms the roof of the carpal tunnel. This space contains *nine* tendons and *one* nerve:

    1) The superficialis and profundus tendons to the fingers.
    2) The flexor pollicis longus tendon.
    3) The median nerve.

    b. The *ulnar* artery and nerve have a *separate* compartment formed by the *volar* carpal ligament.

    c. Note that the *motor* branch of the median nerve leaves the main trunk at the distal edge of the

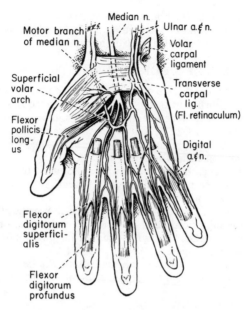

Fig. 5-2.—Palm of hand.

transverse carpal ligament to innervate the thenar muscles and the radial lumbricals.

D. DORSUM OF THE HAND AND WRIST (Fig. 5-3)

1. Note the extensor tendons of the fingers and their insertions at the base of the *middle* phalanges.
2. There are two tendons to the index finger and (with considerable anatomic variation) two tendons to the fifth digit.

E. RADIAL ASPECT OF THE WRIST (Fig. 5-4)

1. This region is injured frequently. The long and short extensor tendons and their insertions and

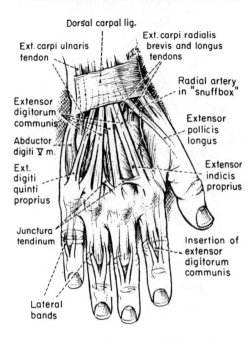

Fig. 5-3.—Dorsum of hand.

the abductor pollicis longus tendon of the thumb are shown.

2. Of greater practical importance is the *sensory* (superficial) branch of the *radial* nerve, frequently overlooked in lacerations of this region.

3. If this structure is *not* repaired, the proximal end forms a neuroma that may become very tender and painful.

4. The extensor carpi radialis longus and brevis are shown. The brevis is *ulnar* to the longus and is the *prime* wrist extensor.

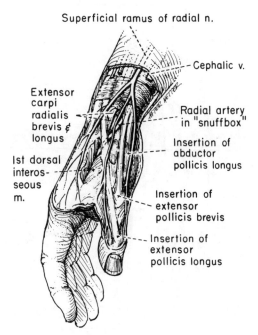

Fig. 5-4.—Superficial ramus of radial n.

F. SENSORY INNERVATION OF THE HAND (Fig. 5-5)

A clear understanding of the sensory innervation of the hand allows an immediate diagnosis of nerve injury to be made simply by using a cotton wisp and then a pin to test the skin surface distal to an injury in the location of a major nerve.

III. DIAGNOSIS

A. Place the patient supine on a cart or table with the arm at a right angle to the body on a sturdy arm board. A Mayo stand or table should be available and covered with sterile towels. The examiner should wear a cap and mask.

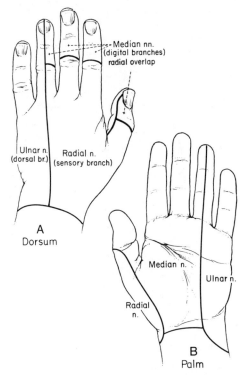

Fig. 5-5.—Sensory innervation of hand.

B. Sterile gloves, towels, hemostats, tissue forceps and several gauze dressings should be on the stand.

C. A very simple chart (Fig. 5-6) should be used to record all findings.
 1. A mirror image allows recording of either surface of both hands.
 2. All abnormalities can be included:
    a. Scars.
    b. The bands, nodules, flexion deformities, etc., of a Dupuytren's contracture.

EXAMINATION OF THE HAND

Name _____   Date _____

Employer _____   Wrist

D/A _____   D. F. __ __   R. D. __ __

Major hand _____   V. F. __ __   U. D. __ __

Injured hand _____   Thumb

Abduction _____

Opposition _____

(Normal-tip touches head of
5th M. C.)

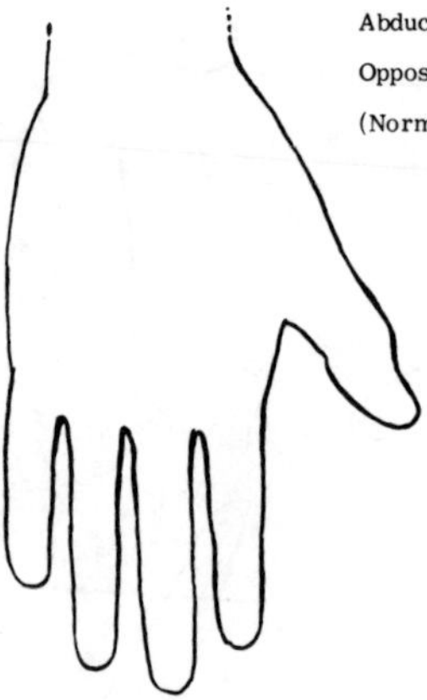

Distance pulp of
finger lacks
of touching
palmar crease = _____ __ __ __ __

Range of Motion of Joints = $\dfrac{\text{Degrees - Extension}}{\text{Degrees - Flexion}}$

Circumference

Sensory impairment indicated by shading

Biceps ___ ___

Grip strength ___ ___   Forearm ___ ___

Fig. 5-6.—Chart for examination of the hand.

    c. Amputations.
    d. Status of the blood supply.
    e. Nerve deficits.
    f. Bone changes (traumatic, congenital).
    g. Tumors.
    h. Tendon injuries; scarring.
    i. Muscle weakness or atrophy.

    j.   Joint changes.
    k.   Infected areas, type, presence of pus, etc.
    l.   Lacerations, bites, etc.

D. TYPES OF INJURIES

1. Vascular Injury.
    a.   A cold, pulseless hand indicates severe arterial damage.
    b.   Circulation must be restored promptly in the main operating suite.
    c.   Significant bleeding can ordinarily be controlled by a compression bandage.
    d.   If bleeding persists, a blood pressure cuff applied to the upper arm and inflated to above the systolic blood pressure will stop or slow the bleeding.
    e.   The cuff must be deflated every 15 minutes to allow full tissue perfusion.

2. Skin Loss.
This usually is apparent immediately upon inspection of the wound and, if at all extensive, will require skin grafting in the main operating suite.

3. Bone Trauma.
The examiner will suspect bone injury if the normal architecture of the hand is distorted. Posteroanterior, oblique, and lateral x-ray films should be ordered.

4. Tendon Injuries.
    a.   Inability to flex the distal phalanx with immobilization of the middle phalanx indicates division of the flexor digitorum profundus (Fig. 5-7).
    b.   Holding all digits in extension except the one injured tests function of the *flexor digitorum superficialis* (Fig. 5-8).
    c.   A laceration over the dorsal surface and inability to extend the digit fully suggests severance of:
        1)   The common extensor tendons.
        2)   The extensor indicis proprius.

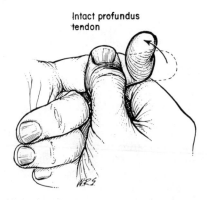

Fig. 5-7.—Testing for flexor digitorum profundus.

Fig. 5-8.—Test for flexor digitorum superficialis.

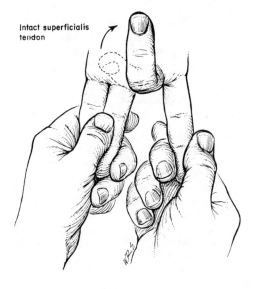

3) The extensor digiti quinti proprius.

d. Lacerations near the distal joint and droop of the distal phalanx indicate injury of the extensor complex in this region (mallet-finger deformity).

e. Inability to extend fully the distal phalanx of the thumb means division of the extensor pollicis longus tendon.

f. Injuries over the *metacarpal of the thumb and the radial aspect of the wrist* with inability to extend and abduct the thumb suggest injuries to the short extensor and long abductor tendons. The long extensor also may be divided.

5. **Wrist Lacerations.**

a. Severe lacerations of the volar surface of the wrist may involve:

1) Radial and ulnar arteries.

2) Median and ulnar nerves.

3) The digital and wrist flexors.

4) The *extent* of the injury *must* be *diagnosed accurately.*

b. Lacerations on dorsum.

1) The integrity of the extensors of the wrist is tested by ability to extend the wrist fully.

2) Intact digital tendons are *synergistic* in this motion and the examiner must ascertain whether the *muscle bellies* of the wrist extensors are contracting.

6. **Nerve Injuries.**

a. Anesthesia distal to lacerations in the digits or palm suggests severance of the *digital sensory* nerves.

b. Severance of the *ulnar* nerve at the wrist causes anesthesia of the ulnar side of the palm, the fifth digit and the ulnar half of the ring digit.

c. The *dorsal* sensory branch of the ulnar nerve leaves the main trunk about 5 cm. proximal to the distal flexion crease of the wrist. (Severance of the ulnar nerve *distal* to the bifurcation still allows the patient to feel pinprick on the dorsum of the hand in the ulnar nerve distribution [a trap for the unwary]).

d. Complete severance of the median nerve of the wrist results in anesthesia of the radial side of the palm, the radial half of the ring and of the entire volar surface of the middle, index and thumb digits.

e. Lacerations of the *thenar area* (often very small) may divide the *motor* branch of the median nerve, which innervates the thenar muscles. With such injury, the patient will be unable to oppose the thumb to the base of the fifth digit well or to abduct it normally.

f. Damage to the *motor* branch of the *ulnar* nerve in the palm will make abduction or adduction of the fingers impossible because of the loss of *interosseous* muscle function.

   1) The best test is to have the patient put his hand palm down on a table and attempt to deviate the *index* finger *radially*.

   2) One may observe and palpate the first dorsal interosseous muscle located on the radial aspect of the second metacarpal bone (dorsum) and assay the extent of movement and muscle tone.

g. Another test for ulnar motor nerve injury is the attempt to pinch strongly between the volar surfaces of the thumb and index digits. In trying to do this, the patient will hyperflex the interphalangeal joint of the thumb (Froment's sign).

h. Lacerations of the radial aspect of the wrist (near the "snuffbox") often divide the *sensory* branch of the *radial* nerve.

   1) Absent or decreased sensation in the distribution of this nerve results.

   2) If the nerve is not repaired, an exquisitely tender neuroma may develop, with associated hypesthesias.

III. NERVE BLOCKS

See Chapter 6, "Adult Regional Anesthesia."

A. GENERAL CONSIDERATIONS

1. Adequate treatment of injuries and infections of the hand is impossible without adequate anesthesia. Nerve blocks in the digits and at the wrist are relatively simple to perform, almost never fail and give complete anesthesia for up to 3 hours.

2. The patient must *always* be asked whether he has ever received local anesthetics and, if so, whether a systemic reaction to them has occurred.

   a. If the patient has a positive history of allergy to local anesthetics, their use is *contraindicated* and a general anesthetic will be required.

   b. If the patient has never received local anesthetics, or does not remember receiving them, one must be extremely cautious if such a patient also has a strong allergic history or is extremely apprehensive.

3. As a rule, digital nerve blocks can be used in children; wrist blocks are more difficult because of fear and lack of cooperation. The *advantage* of the local anesthetic is that it may be administered whether or not the patient has recently ingested food or liquid.

4. Injection of local anesthetics *directly* into a wound for debridement and repair *obscures* the normal anatomy and is potentially dangerous, since it may *spread infection.*

B. DIGITAL NERVE BLOCK (Fig. 5-9)

1. Several techniques for digital nerve block are employed. However, antiseptic solutions containing adrenalin should *never* be used, except in the most expert hands. Adrenalin may cause severe vasoconstriction, resulting in gangrene and necessitating eventual amputation of the digit.

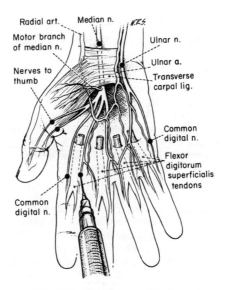

Fig. 5-9.—Sites for nerve blocks.

2. We instill the solution for digital nerve block *prior* to final preparation for operation (after preliminary cleansing) to ensure thorough, pain-free final preparation.

   a. The surgeon dons sterile gloves and places the patient's hand on a sterile towel with the palm up.

   b. A disposable syringe is filled with 10 ml. of 1% solution of lidocaine (Xylocaine) hydrochloride. Other anesthetic agents may be used; procaine is not recommended because of its short duration.

   c. A no. 25 hypodermic needle, 3/4 inch length, is fitted on the syringe.

   d. The needle point is placed slightly below the edge of the digital cleft and angled 20 degrees from the long axis of the digit being anesthetized.

e. The needle is inserted slowly until it encounters the proximal phalanx. It is then withdrawn slightly and the plunger is pulled back to be sure that the needle point is not in a vessel.

f. Three milliliters of solution are then injected, producing "ballooning" of the web space. The procedure is then repeated through a separate needle puncture on the other side of the digit.

g. For the fifth digit, the solution is placed just proximal to its base, 5 mm. from the ulnar border of the hand.

h. For the index digit, radial side, the solution is placed proximal to the proximal flexion crease, 5 mm. ulnar to the radial aspect of the hand (volar surface).

i. The digital nerves of the thumb flank the flexor pollicis longus tendon. Injection of 2-3 ml. of solution is performed on each side of the tendon at the base of the thumb.

j. If an injury affects the dorsum of the finger or edges up onto the lateral borders, it is advisable to supplement these blocks with field blocks on the dorsum of the digit above the clefts. Two milliliters of solution are placed transversely across the dorsum of the digit.

3. After instillation of these blocks, final preparation and draping of the hand is performed, allowing the anesthetic time to "set."

a. The hand is then elevated for 5 minutes and a no. 8 French catheter is placed around the base of the finger and held with a medium-sized hemostat (Fig. 5-10).

b. *Rubber bands are never used,* because they may be forgotten and incorporated into the bandage, producing gangrene and necessitating amputation. It is almost impossible to overlook a long catheter held in place with a hemostat.

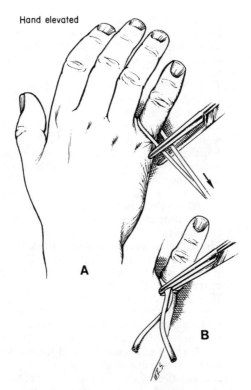

Hand elevated

A

B

Fig. 5-10.—Obtaining a bloodless field in a digit.

C. NERVE BLOCKS AT THE WRIST

1. Median Nerve Block.

If the palmaris longus tendon is present, the needle placement is to its radial side just proximal to the distal flexion crease of the wrist.

a. The needle is angled slightly ulnarward and often a slight "give" can be felt as the needle point penetrates the superficial fascia.

    b. Paresthesias in the distribution of the median nerve are often elicited as the needle point contacts the nerve.

    c. It is preferable to inject the anesthetic *around* the nerve, since intraneural injections may produce a troublesome neuritis.

    d. If the palmaris longus tendon is absent, the solution is injected about 1 cm. ulnar to the flexor carpi radialis tendon.

    e. Five milliliters of solution is injected, with care taken to avoid vascular structures.

    f. The needle is then withdrawn to a subcutaneous position and the remaining subcutaneous tissues across the wrist (palmar cutaneous branch) are infiltrated with the remaining 5 ml. of solution.

2. Ulnar Nerve Block.

    a. The ulnar nerve lies quite superficial, just to the radial side of the *pisiform* bone, which is easily palpated. The needle is directed to this location and 3-5 ml. of solution is injected.

3. Radial Nerve Block at the Wrist.

The radial nerve lies near the cephalic vein at the proximal portion of the "snuffbox." Injecting this area with 5 ml. of solution anesthetizes the sensory branch of the radial nerve.

4. Ulnar Nerve Block for the Dorsum of the Hand.

The dorsum is anesthetized by a field block on the dorsum just distal to the ulna. Five ml. of solution is injected subcutaneously from the mid-portion of the dorsum of the wrist to its ulnar side.

5. Ulnar Nerve Block at the Elbow.

The ulnar nerve lies quite superficial in the epicondylar notch at the ulnar aspect of the elbow. Five ml. of solution injected in this area provides satisfactory ulnar nerve block.

6. **Axillary Nerve Block.**
   a. Axillary, brachial plexus and double tourniquet intravenous blocks should be done by an experienced anesthesiologist. They are described in detail in Chapter 6, "Adult Regional Anesthesia."
   b. These blocks, if done well, are most useful. They eliminate or minimize pain of the hemostatic tourniquet.
   c. Sedation can be given as needed.
   d. *All* of these should be done in the main operating suite.

IV. WOUND PREPARATION

A. The patient is taken immediately into an examination room and the injured hand is immersed in a basin filled with warm water and soap or an antiseptic solution. Superficial dirt is soaked away and the patient benefits psychologically from this preliminary treatment.

B. For definitive wound preparation, see Chapter 2, section on "Preparation of Wound."

V. HEMOSTATIC TOURNIQUET

A. Repair of even minor wounds is facilitated by the use of an arm tourniquet.

B. A tourniquet should not be used unless the surgeon is familiar with the dangers involved. Very high pressures can be applied accidentally if the gauge is faulty. The tourniquet becomes very painful after 30-45 minutes unless the area proximal to it has been anesthetized.

C. The arm tourniquet should be used with *every* major procedure in the main operating room.
   1. Pressure should be regulated to 50 mm. Hg above the systolic, but must not exceed 250 mm. Hg for adults and 150-200 mm. Hg for children.

D. Tourniquet use *should not* exceed 1½ hours. If more time is needed, the tourniquet is released and the

extremity allowed to perfuse for 20 minutes before re-
application.

VI. TREATMENT

A. LACERATIONS

1. **The Cardinal Principles of Management:**
   a. Strict asepsis.
   b. Excision of the traumatized *skin margins* and all
       loose or devitalized tissue.
   c. Closure without tension. See Chapter 4 for man-
       agement of contused, stellate and slicing wounds
       and the recommended suture materials.
   d. Primary suture is *not* recommended for:
       1) Wounds seen more than 8 hours after injury.
       2) Significant skin loss, since grafting will be
          needed.
       3) Human and animal bites. (Animal bites seen
          promptly that are *not* punctures may be
          closed primarily.)
       4) Puncture wounds.
   e. Exposed tendon or bone with soft-tissue loss
       usually requires coverage with some type of pedi-
       cle flap. Such procedures demand expert judg-
       ment and technique and must be performed in
       the main operating suite.

B. FINGER TIP INJURIES

1. Most injuries and infections in the hand occur in the
   finger tips. Early wound closure with the least possible deformity is the prime objective.
2. The injuries vary from simple lacerations to avulsions
   of skin and soft tissue. Tendon and bone may be
   exposed.
3. Complicated operations to restore pulp tissue and
   sensation are often better done as *secondary* procedures.
4. Attempts to rehabilitate the *index* digit may be

difficult if the middle digit is uninjured, since the patient tends to use the latter instead of working at rehabilitating the index digit.

5. The *thumb* is the most important digit of the hand, and special effort must be directed at preservation of length, adequate pulp tissue and good sensation.

6. **Types of Coverage.**

   a. In general, intermediate-thickness skin grafts are the simplest and most practical. Their use, however, is contraindicated over exposed tendon or bone.

   b. The cross-finger pedicle flap can be used for primary closure. Prime indications are:
      1) Loss of pulp tissue.
      2) Preservation of length.

   c. When full-thickness tissue loss is extensive, body pedicle flaps may be necessary.

   d. Neurovascular island pedicle flaps can be used *secondarily* to improve sensation.

C. TRAUMATIC AMPUTATIONS

1. **Tips of Digits.**

   a. Attempting to replace amputated finger tips is *not advisable* in adults because such tissue rarely survives. Replacement of a cleanly amputated short segment, however, may be attempted in an infant or child.

   b. When the dorsum of the tip is involved, if a reasonable amount of the fingernail is intact, it should *not* be removed, nor should the delicate skin at the base of the nail be damaged to avoid interference with new nail growth.

   c. The fingernail remnant can be used in anchoring a skin graft and also acts as a splint to the tip.

   d. Blood which has accumulated under the nail should be evacuated through a small hole.

   e. If one neurovascular pedicle is intact, the tip will survive.

    f. If the tip amputation is oblique, it may be possible to close it primarily by removing part of the distal phalanx.

    g. Because the *thumb is a prime digit,* preservation of length with a pain-free, well-cushioned tip is necessary. Exposed bone should be covered with adjacent soft tissue and a skin graft. A cross-finger pedicle flap may be necessary.

    h. Preservation of length in the index digit is also important. If the amputation is through the distal interphalangeal joint, the head of the middle phalanx should be tapered and the wound closed primarily without tension on the skin flaps.

    i. Some of the bone in the remaining digits may be removed to permit primary closure. If this is not possible, the end of the bone should be covered by soft tissue and a skin graft applied.

D. AVULSIONS

1. Avulsion wounds are characterized by the tearing of skin and soft tissue from the deeper structures.
    a. Although the arterial supply may appear satisfactory, venous return may be badly damaged, especially with *distally* based flaps.
    b. If the edges of the flaps show a poor blood supply, they should be removed and the gap covered by a skin graft.

E. BITES AND PUNCTURE WOUNDS

1. Human bites are especially likely to become infected and usually are sustained over the metacarpophalangeal joint.
2. They frequently involve the extensor tendon mechanism, joint capsule, and the joint itself.
3. The wounds *should not* be closed. The skin around the wound is cleaned thoroughly and the wound thoroughly irrigated.
4. A bulky dressing should be applied to the entire hand.

5. Antibiotics are *indicated* (Part I, "Antibiotics in the Emergency Service").

6. Puncture wounds caused by animal bites, thin knives or ice picks are treated in the same manner.

F. WRINGER AND ROLLER INJURIES

1. Severe injury is obvious and the skin is usually badly damaged especially if it has been subjected to the shearing effect of turning rollers.

2. The *danger* is in underestimating what appears to be a minor injury.

   a. Should hemorrhage occur in the muscles, ischemia, necrosis and subsequent Volkmann's contracture may result in a *permanently* disabled extremity.

   b. Wringer injuries should be cleansed thoroughly and the entire hand and arm enclosed in a resilient compression dressing with elevation of the extremity.

   c. X-ray films must be obtained.

   d. *All* children with wringer injuries should be hospitalized, if only for a relatively short time, to be sure there are no complications.

G. TENDON AND NERVE INJURIES (Fig. 5-11)

1. Satisfactory repair of tendon and nerve injuries requires:

   a. The facilities of the main operating suite.

   b. Competent assistance.

   c. Excellent anesthesia.

   d. Most important, the skill of a surgeon experienced in the management of these injuries.

H. DRESSING AND SPLINTS

1. Wounds of the Hand or Wrist.

   a. After wound closure, sterile nylon or fine-mesh gauze is applied, with several sterile gauze squares then placed over it.

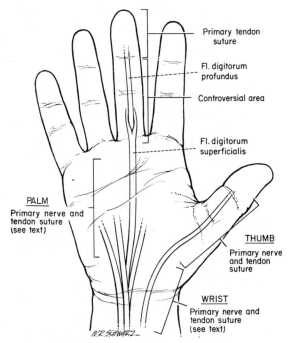

Fig. 5-11.—Areas of primary nerve and tendon suture (see text).

   b. Additional gauze squares are placed in each inter-
      digital cleft to:
      1) Absorb perspiration.
      2) Prevent compression of the digital neurovas-
         cular bundles.
      3) Avoid skin maceration.
   c. More gauze squares are fluffed and applied
      around all sides of the hand and forearm to form
      a bulky dressing.
   d. If the injury does *not* involve the finger tips, they
      are left exposed in order to assay the circulation
      and sensation postoperatively.

    e. The gauze squares are held in place by a gauze roll (Kling). If additional padding is necessary for plaster splints, 3-inch Webril is applied.

    f. The hand is then splinted in a functional position:

       1) The wrist in 20 degrees of dorsiflexion.

       2) Each digit in a gentle, semiflexed position.

       3) The thumb in *abduction* and *opposition*.

    g. A plaster splint of 12-14 thicknesses of 3-4-inch wide strips is then applied and molded to the volar aspect of the palm and forearm. Cohesive works very well in holding the plaster splint and dressing in place.

2. **Wounds of the Digits.**

    a. The same general principles apply to dressing of individual digits.

    b. *Immobilization* promotes wound healing.

    c. If a laceration is confined to a digit, a foam-rubber, aluminum splint should be applied with the digit in semiflexion.

3. **Follow-up Care.**

    a. If a wound has been prepared thoroughly, debrided and sutured with *meticulous* technique, the initial dressing may be left in place for 7-10 days.

    b. If there is any risk of infection or other complication, the extremity should be inspected the following day.

    c. Sutures should not be removed too soon.

       1) Since palmar skin is thick and heals slowly, sutures should be left for 2-3 weeks.

       2) The skin of the dorsum of the hand and forearm heals more quickly and sutures may be removed in 10-14 days.

VII. INFECTIONS

A. GENERAL CONSIDERATIONS

1. Significant numbers of patients with acute hand infections come to the Emergency Service for treatment.
2. Trauma to the hand is the most common industrial injury, with infection a frequent sequela.
3. Children are especially susceptible to infections following injury, as are butchers and meat handlers.
4. Hospital personnel are subject to infections from contaminated needles, etc., and present a particular problem in treatment because of resistant organisms and hepatitis.
5. Immediate decision is necessary as to whether adequate treatment requires use of the main operating suite.
6. *Infections* should be examined and treated in a room adequately equipped and used *only* for that purpose. Such rooms must be thoroughly cleaned after each treatment.
7. *Pitting edema* of the dorsum of the hand is characteristic of almost all significant hand infections. Rarely does the dorsum contain localized pus.

B. GENERAL TREATMENT PRINCIPLES

Treatment of the infected hand includes the following:
1. *Immobilization* to ensure rest, achieved with bulky dressings and a plaster splint which extends from the finger tips to the upper forearm. The wrist should be dorsiflexed and the fingers naturally flexed with the thumb in abduction and opposition.
2. *Elevation* to prevent or reduce swelling.
   a. When the patient is up and about, a sling is employed in which the hand points toward the opposite shoulder.
   b. When he is in bed, the extremity should be elevated on two or three pillows or suspended with

the forearm pointing straight up and the upper
arm supported.

3. *Gram stain, culture and sensitivity studies* of pus or
exudate.

4. *Antibiotic therapy,* to abort early diffuse infection
or hasten recovery in established infections.

5. *Tetanus* prophylaxis (Chap. 7).

6. *Drainage* of localized abscesses through properly
placed incisions.

C. DIFFUSE (EARLY-STAGE) LESIONS

1. The patient usually *presents* with throbbing pain
and swelling of the hand or digit of 1 or 2 days'
duration.

2. *Examination* may reveal local or generalized swelling,
pain, tenderness, cellulitis and lymphangitis or enlarged epitrochlear or axillary lymph glands.

3. A wound of entry may be present. The important
feature is the *absence* of localized pus.

4. Incision in the early lesion is *contraindicated* unless
there is absolute evidence of pus.

5. If the presence of pus is questionable, 2 or 3 ml. of
saline should be injected and aspirated; culture of
this fluid and the needle tip may afford positive
identification of the organism.

6. The streptococcus is the usual offender. Large doses
of procaine penicillin G are given intramuscularly.

7. *Bed rest,* with *immobilization* and *elevation* of the
affected extremity, is prescribed.

8. Frequent re-examination is necessary. If the infection has not been aborted, incision and drainage are
indicated after the infection has localized.

9. Warm moist soaks are not ordinarily used.

D. LOCALIZED LESIONS

1. The pain pattern differs in that there is usually a 4-5-
day history of pain and swelling.

2. The patient is placed supine on the operating table
with the arm extended on a sturdy armstand.

3. The patient must be asked about sensitivity to penicillin *prior* to its administration.
   a. Patients with penicillin sensitivity or a strong allergic background are given erythromycin, 100 mg. I.M.
   b. Hospital employees or patients in whom a penicillin resistant organism is strongly suspected are given oxacillin, etc. (see Part 1, "Antibiotics in the Emergency Service").
4. *Procaine penicillin G* or another antibiotic is given by I.M. at least 30 minutes before incision and drainage.
5. The area of maximum tenderness or visible pus is noted.
6. After *preliminary* preparation of the hand, a wrist or digital nerve block is instilled.
7. After *onset* of anesthesia, *definitive preparation* of the extremity is performed.

E. INCISIONS—GENERAL PRINCIPLES

1. Small incisions are placed directly over the area of maximum tenderness or visible pus and follow the normal skin lines.
2. Digital and palmar skin creases are *never* crossed by vertical incisions. Transverse, diagonal or curving incisions are used.
3. Specimens of pus are taken for *gram stain, culture* and sensitivity studies. The abscess cavity is then thoroughly swabbed.
4. The wound is explored with a blunt probe if a sinus tract is suspected.
5. If a bone is felt to be roughened, it probably is also infected.
6. "Packing" of abscess cavities is absolutely *contraindicated.*
7. A small ellipse of skin is removed to afford adequate drainage.
8. A bulky dressing and sling are applied.
9. The initial dressing change is performed on the following day.

10. If *throbbing pain* is still present, the initial incision may have been inadequate and must be enlarged. Another intramuscular dose of the antibiotic is given.
11. If the pain is subsiding, less frequent dressing changes are needed and early movement of the affected part is encouraged.
12. Delayed healing may result from:
    a. Retained foreign body.
    b. Pre-existing degenerative arthritis.
    c. Septic arthritis.
    d. Resistance of the bacteria to the antibiotic.

F. SPECIFIC LESIONS

1. **Pulp Abscess** (Fig. 5-12).
   a. The infection often is located in the terminal, volar pulp space (felon).
   b. It also may be located over the middle or proximal phalanges.
   c. Typically after localization there is pain, swelling, discoloration and induration.
   d. *INCISIONS* for drainage are placed as indicated above after intramuscular injection of antibiotics.

Fig. 5-12.—Pulp abscess.

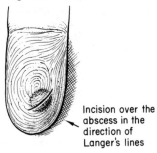

Incision over the abscess in the direction of Langer's lines

Incision for drainage of a pulp abscess

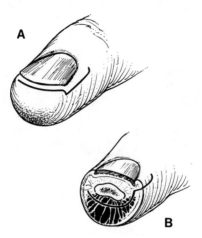

Fig. 5-13.—Incision for a felon.

The old through-and-through incision is *contraindicated* (Fig. 5-13).

2. **Paronychia.**
   a. Acute paronychia is an infection of the digit that begins in the skin around the fingernail. It is frequently caused by the patient picking at a "hangnail."
   b. Paronychia may be acute or chronic, with or without subungual extension.
   c. If the lesion is confined to the skin, it is unroofed and drained.
   d. If pus is present under the *base of the nail,* the skin is gently pushed proximalward and the base is elevated in its entire width and removed (Fig. 5-14).
   e. If the distal portion of the nail is unaffected, it is *not* removed. *No* incisions are required.
   f. Chronic paronychia is often due to:
      1) Neglected acute infections.

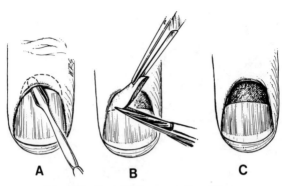

Fig. 5-14.—Draining for pus at the nail base.

    2) A fungus.
    3) Frequent immersion in water.
  g. **Treatment** is directed toward keeping the finger
     dry, checking for fungus infection and prescrib-
     ing the indicated medication.

3. **Web Space Infections.**
  a. These infections are situated in the fatty tissue
    of the distal palm in the interdigital clefts.
  b. Examination reveals erythema, pain, swelling
    and tenderness. The involved digits may be held
    in abduction but can be flexed and extended
    without great pain.
  c. The presence of localized pus may be quite diffi-
    cult to detect. Again, needle aspiration may be
    useful.
  d. **Treatment.**
    After preparation, nerve block and administra-
    tion of an antibiotic,
     1) A short transverse incision is made in the
      palm proximal to the affected web.
     2) The cavity is carefully cleaned and explored
      to detect any sinus tract to the dorsum.

4. **Palmar Abscesses.**

    a. These infections usually are deep to the palmar fascia. They may occur in conjunction with an *acute suppurative tenosynovitis.*

    b. The abscess may be confined to the thenar space or the middle palmar space and, if so, drainage is directed to the specific area involved.

    c. *Examination of the hand* will show:
        1) Marked swelling.
        2) Digits held relatively immobile.
        3) Extremely tender, red or purple skin.
        4) Pitting edema of the dorsum in most cases.
        5) Usually, fever and lymph gland enlargement.

    d. **Treatment** of the deep palmar abscess is a serious matter that usually requires *full* operating facilities including a hemostatic tourniquet.
        1) *Drainage* technique must be meticulous. Incisions are carefully placed to avoid injury to tendons, nerves and vessels. Incisions are usually curving or transverse.
        2) Neglected palmar abscesses may cause severe compression of the median nerve and extend proximalward to the ulnar or radial bursa. *Decompression* of the affected structures is indicated.

5. **Septic Arthritis.**

    a. The lesion is an infected wound over the dorsum of the metacarpophalangeal or interphalangeal joint, with pain, swelling and tenderness of the entire digit.

    b. A sinus tract may exist.

    c. Flexion and extension of the joint produce extreme pain.

    d. X-rays of the affected areas should be taken.

    e. The involved joint should be explored and thoroughly cleansed.

    f. Immobilization, antibiotic therapy and frequent dressing changes are needed to avoid full-blown osteomyelitis with bone and joint destruction.

6. **Acute Suppurative Tenosynovitis** (Fig. 5-15).
    a. The usual findings are:
        1) Diffuse swelling and erythema of the involved digit.
        2) Fusiform swelling of the digit.
        3) Digit held in flexion.
        4) Exquisite pain elicited by *passive* flexion and extension.
        5) Tenderness localized over the tendon sheath elicited by light pressure with a closed hemostat.
    b. Pus in the tendon sheath with or without proximal extension must be drained in the main operating suite.
        1) General anesthesia or brachial-plexus or axillary block and a hemostatic tournique are employed.

Fig. 5-15.—Drainage and irrigation of an acute tenosynovitis.

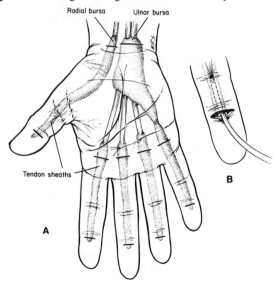

Radial bursa   Ulnar bursa

Tendon sheaths

A   B

2) The classic midlateral incision is no longer the procedure of choice.

3) A transverse incision is made at the site of the puncture wound or obvious abscess, or just *distal* to the *distal interphalangeal joint,* (Fig. 5-15).

4) After the infected sheaths have been opened, a fine ureteric or polyethylene catheter is used to irrigate them with a saline or penicillin solution—until all pus has been removed.

5) The edges of the skin incisions are *excised* to ensure adequate drainage.

6) A very fine catheter may be left in place for 24 or 48 hours for intermittent injection of a solution containing polymyxin B sulfate and bacitracin.

7) Evidence of pus *proximally* in the palm, wrist or forearm requires drainage of these areas as well.

8) Local irrigation with antibiotics is supplemented with their massive systemic administration.

9) The patient is *hospitalized.*

7. **Boils and Carbuncles.**
   a. The usual location of these lesions is the dorsum.
   b. Their appearance is characteristic and incision
   . and drainage are *not indicated* as they almost always respond to adequate penicillin therapy, immobilization and elevation. A subcuticular lesion can be opened without anesthesia to facilitate drainage.

8. **Less Common Lesions Included in the Differential Diagnosis:**
   a. Erysipeloid.—Occurring mainly in butchers and fish handlers, this is a well-differentiated, purplish lesion.
   b. Herpes simplex (Herpetic whitlow).—Physicians, dentists and nurses are most often affected.

      a) The lesion has the appearance of a pulp infection but vesicles soon appear.

      b) Bacterial culture is negative but virus particles can be demonstrated in the exudate.

c. Barber's hand.—The infection is caused by hairs penetrating the finger webs. The treatment is directed at the superimposed infection.

d. Grease- or paint-gun injuries.—These lesions are caused by injection under high pressure of grease, paint or other foreign substances. *Treatment* is early and thorough decompression in the main operating suite.

e. Gout.—When this condition affects the digits, signs and symptoms may mimic a pulp infection or septic arthritis. The serum uric acid usually is elevated.

f. Metastatic tumors.

      1) Primary tumors of the hand, except for those on the skin, are rare.

      2) Metastatic lesions may be mistaken for infections.

      3) A proper history and x-ray films will disclose the correct diagnosis.

g. Malignant melanoma.

      1) The most common location is under the fingernail.

      2) The first sign usually is a painless, dark brown or black spot visible under the distal edge of the nail. It may become secondarily infected.

      3) Any dark spot under the nail which persists should be removed by excisional biopsy.

      4) Discoloration may not be present.

      5) A persistent, small ulcer is an indication for excisional biopsy.

h. Pyogenic granuloma.—The typical lesion is a raspberry-like structure often following chronic infection.

      1) It is benign and, if small, may be treated by repeated cautery.

      2) If larger, it should be excised.

i. Glomus tumor.
    1) The patient presents with severe tenderness
       in the end of a digit.
    2) Pain is brought on by light touch or exposure
       to heat or cold.
    3) The tumor is very small, usually subungual
       and pigmented.
    4) The lesion may *extend* volarward through
       the distal phalanx and into the volar pulp
       space.
    5) Complete local excision relieves the symp-
       toms.

CHAPTER 6

Adult Regional Anesthesia in the Emergency Service

REUBEN C. BALAGOT, M.D., *and*
VALERIE R. BANDELIN, M.D.

I. INTRODUCTION

A. Patients requiring emergency surgery under general anesthesia often:
   1. Have eaten recently and are subject to the danger of vomiting and aspiration.
   2. Cannot be worked up thoroughly and may suffer from chronic illnesses that make general anesthesia hazardous.
   3. Are taking medications which will affect both anesthesia and their underlying status adversely.

B. The anesthetist is limited to drugs which minimize hazards and complications.

C. Regional (local) anesthesia, therefore, becomes ideal for the Emergency Service patient.

D. This discussion will concern only those procedures that are relatively easy to perform and that minimize hazardous physiologic changes.

E. Since, under certain circumstances, using regional anesthesia is unwise or impossible, methods, techniques and choice of agents for *general* anesthesia are briefly described.

II. REGIONAL ANESTHESIA

A. LOCAL INFILTRATION BLOCKS

1. This probably is the type used most frequently.
2. The surgeon or anesthetist must know his drugs and their side effects thoroughly and how to treat untoward reactions.
3. It is not desirable to inject local anesthetics *into* a wound if it is possible to obtain anesthesia some other way.
4. Proximal and, if possible, distal nerve blocks are much superior.
5. "Field" blocks can be most useful if skillfully performed.
6. To infiltrate around a wound:
   a. Raise a small skin wheal with a 1/2-inch, 25- or 30-gauge needle.
   b. After a short wait, insert the block needle through it.
   c. A 10-ml. Luer-lock syringe and a 2.5- or 3-inch 22-gauge needle is needed.
   d. Inject the drug as close to the dermis as possible.
   e. Inserting the needle to its full length and *then* injecting the drug as the needle is withdrawn is good technique.
   f. Repeat this step until the entire area has been injected.
   g. *Wait* until the anesthetic takes effect. Jabbing the skin every 30 seconds produces pain and increases apprehension.
   h. A 0.5% solution of lidocaine (Xylocaine), hydrochloride, mepivacaine, carbocaine, etc., is *sufficient* and increases the volume that may be used without appreciably increasing toxicity.
7. Sedating the patient carefully is wise, since every injured patient is having pain and is frightened.
   a. Meperidine (Demerol) combined with promethazine (Phenergan), a mild tranquilizer, works well, minimizing nausea and enhancing sedation.

1) The narcotic may be easily reversed by a suitable antagonist at any time.
2) *Dosage* for the average adult:
   a) Meperidine, 50-150 mg., in increments of 25-50 mg., I.V., with promethazine 25-50 mg.

B. FIELD BLOCKS

1. As the name indicates, these differ from local infiltration blocks in that much larger areas can be anesthetized.
2. Infiltrate each anatomical layer beginning with the skin.
3. It is mandatory to *cross the nerve supply* of the area to be anesthetized.
   a. An example is the technique that allows repair of a large wound of the anterior abdomen from the xiphoid to the umbilicus.
   b. Infiltrate layer by layer starting from just above the xiphoid.
   c. Slant downward and laterally along the costal arch.
   d. Then, angle caudally to the level of the antero-superior iliac spine.
   e. This block affords anesthesia down to the peritoneum and is ideal for the critically ill or debilitated patient.
   f. A drawback is the rather large quantity of anesthetic needed.

C. REGIONAL NERVE BLOCKS

See Chapter 5, "Injuries and Infections of the Hand."

1. **Head and Neck.**
   a. Intra-oral blocks:
      1) The trigeminal nerve and branches.
         a) Mandibular nerve.
            i) Mental nerve.
            ii) Inferior alveolar nerve.

          iii) Lingual nerve.

          iv) Maxillary, infraorbital branch.

  2) The mandibular nerve.

    a) Inject at the angle of the mandible posterior to the last molar.

    b) Paresthesias of the tongue (lingual nerve) or the lower jaw (inferior alveolar nerve) are frequent.

    c) Dosage: 2-4 ml. of a 2% solution.

  3) The mental nerve.

    a) Supplies sensation to the anterior aspect of the jaw.

    b) Inject at the gingivobuccal margin on a line between the premolars.

  4) The infra-orbital (branch of the maxillary).

    a) Inject through the mucosa above the upper premolar.

  5) Dosage: 2-4 ml. of a 2% solution.

  6) Extra-oral blocks are possible but *not* recommended.

b. *Extra-oral blocks.*

  1) Supra-orbital and supratrochlear divisions of the *opthalmic nerve.*

  2) Location: medial aspect of the orbital ridge just above the inner canthus.

  3) Administer block at this location.

  4) Provides anesthesia for forehead and anterior one-half of scalp.

  5) The lateral orbital nerve may be blocked at the upper, outer aspect of the orbital ridge above the outer canthus.

c. *Deep and superficial cervical plexus.*

  1) The deep cervical-plexus block is simple but requires instruction and experience.

  2) The superficial cervical plexus is:

    a) Very accessible at the posterior margin of the sternocleidomastoid muscle midway between the origin and the insertion.

    b) Injection of 10-15 ml. of a 1.0% or 1.5% local anesthetic will provide anesthesia for skin, muscle and subcutaneous tissues of the front of the neck and the anterior aspect of the chest almost down to the nipple line.

2. **Upper Extremities** (see Chap. 5).
    a. *Axillary block.*
        1) For details, the reader is referred to the section on pediatric anesthesia (Chap. 22).
        2) Although the procedure is the same, there is more tissue over the axillary artery and main nerves.
        3) The nerves are larger with heavier myelinization.
        4) A 3/4- or 1-1/4-inch, 25-gauge needle is more effective in probing for the radial nerve, which may lie deep behind the axillary artery.
        5) *More* anesthetic is needed.
            a) We use a 1-1/2 or 2% concentration of mepivacaine or lidocaine with 1:200,000 epinephrine added to it.
            b) About 7-10 ml. is instilled for every paresthesia.
            c) Up to 30 ml. of a 2% solution can be used. This may be repeated in 30-40 minutes, but a smaller dose is advisable.
    b. *Intravenous lidocaine or mepivacaine.*
        1) Intravenous lidocaine (Xylocaine) anesthesia is described in the section on pediatric anesthesia (Chap. 22).
        2) As long as there are no large tissue gaps which might prevent the anesthetic from diffusing through the veins, it is very useful for adults.
            a) A 20- or 18-gauge plastic needle is put in a vein on the dorsum of the hand.
            b) Infusion of 5% dextrose in water (5% D/W) in a 250-ml. bottle is started.
            c) The injection site on the I.V. set is used for injection.
            d) The needle is taped well down to the hand

and the I.V. tube clamped close to the injection site.

e) A *double-cuffed tourniquet* is placed on the upper arm just below the deltoid.

f) The arm is emptied of blood with an Esmarch or elastic bandage starting from the finger tips up to the tourniquet.

g) The proximal (upper) cuff of the tourniquet is then inflated to a pressure of 250 mm. Hg.

h) Xylocaine, 50 ml. of a 1/2% solution is injected into the I.V. tubing.

i) The I.V. needle is removed; bleeding is controlled with pressure.

j) After 10 minutes, the distal (lower) cuff is *inflated* and the proximal cuff *deflated*.

k) The inflated portion of the cuff is now over an anesthetized area, diminishing the patient's discomfort.

l) It is safe to keep the cuff inflated up to 90 minutes.

m) In prolonged surgical procedures, the needle is left in place and Xylocaine is injected as needed.

n) Mepivacaine in the same concentration can be used but is more irritating to the venous system than Xylocaine.

o) The original method utilized procaine, which has the advantage of low toxicity due to rapid metabolism by pseudocholinesterase in the blood stream. Xylocaine and mepivacaine are both metabolized only in the liver.

3. **Epidural Anesthesia.**

a. This and caudal and spinal anesthetics should be given by a trained anesthetist in the *main operating suite*.

b. We utilize a Tuohy spinal needle with the point rounded so that the likelihood of penetrating the spinal canal is minimized.

4. **Caudal Anesthesia.**
   a. Anatomic variations of the sacrum can cause difficulty in locating the sacral hiatus.
   b. The caudal canal is a part of the epidural space.

5. **Spinal Anesthesia.**
   a. This procedure is easier than the epidural since most physicians have done a few intrathecal or spinal punctures.
   b. It is one step farther than a spinal puncture.
   c. For brief procedures, procaine, 5%, is the anesthetic of choice.
   d. The usual anesthetic used for spinal anesthesia is tetracaine.
      1) This comes in 20-mg. ampules and can be made either *hyperbaric* (heavier than spinal fluid) with 10% dextrose-in-water or *hypobaric* by dissolving it in double distilled sterile water to a concentration of 0.3%.

6. **Chest and Abdomen.**
   a. *Intercostal nerve block* (See Chap. 8, "Thoracic Injuries").
   b. *Paravertebral somatic nerve blocks.*
      1) There are several methods of performing this block, but our preference is to approach the nerve as it comes out through the *intervertebral foramen.*
      2) A skin wheal is raised about 1-1/2-2 cm. lateral to the mid-line opposite a vertebral spine.
      3) A 3-inch, 20-gauge needle is inserted through the wheal until bone is contacted, which should be a lamina.
      4) The needle is then "walked off" laterally until it slips over bone and enters the intervertebral foramen.
      5) After aspiration for blood or spinal fluid, 3-5 ml. of a 1-1/2% local anesthetic are injected.
      6) At the level of the intervertebral foramina, most

of the spinal nerves are in the same fascial plane. It is therefore possible to affect several nerves by injecting greater volumes of local anesthetic at 2- or 3-segment intervals from each other.

7) In the *chest,* this form of block also affects the sympathetic ganglion as it lies in close proximity to the spinal nerve in the intervertebral foramen.

7. The Lower Extremities.

a. *Sciatic-femoral nerve blocks.*

1) The sciatic nerve is approached from a point located 1 inch below the mid-point of a line drawn from the posterior superior iliac spine to the upper border of the greater trochanter.

2) It is a large nerve, and 7-10 ml. of a 1-1/2% anesthetic is used.

3) A 20- or 22-gauge, 3- or 4-inch needle should be used since the nerve is somewhat deep.

4) Paresthesias to the foot should be elicited, otherwise the attempted block will be a failure.

5) The posterior aspect of the thigh, the calf, the foot and nearly up to or just below the knee should be anesthetized.

6) To block the interior aspect of the thigh, a femoral nerve block is needed.

7) The point of entry is located about an inch below the inguinal ligament and just lateral to the *femoral artery.*

a) Paresthesias are rarely elicited for this type of block; therefore volume is needed.

b) About 5-10 ml. of a 1-1/2% solution is injected in a fan-wise manner laterally from the artery, because at this point, the femoral nerve tends to divide quickly into its many branches.

b. *Posterior tibial nerve blocks.*

1) The posterior tibial nerve block covers the

            plantar surface of the foot up to the great
            toe.
        2) The nerve is approached behind the medial
            malleolus in front of the Achilles tendon.
        3) Paresthesias occasionally are elicited.
        4) Five ml. of a 1-1/2% solution of mepivacaine
            is injected.

III. COMPLICATIONS OF REGIONAL ANESTHESIA

A. The regional anesthetic procedures described were se-
    lected primarily on the basis of simplicity of technique
    and easy accessibility of the nerve involved.

B. Except for the intercostal and paravertebral somatic
    nerve blocks, during which inadvertent entry into the
    thoracic cavity possibly causing a pneumothorax and in-
    advertent entry into the intrathecal space through a *pro-
    longed dural sleeve* may cause *massive* anesthesia, most
    of the regional procedures described were selected be-
    cause complications arising from the procedure itself or
    technique involved are usually minimal.

C. *No attempt* will be made to list the management of these
    complications except as they relate to *resuscitation* which
    involves:
    1. Respiratory.
    2. Cardiovascular.
    3. Support and maintenance of the central nervous sys-
       tem (CNS) functions.

D. TOXIC REACTIONS

    1. *Systemic reactions* may well be the most serious com-
       plication of regional anesthetic blocks.
    2. They usually are associated with inadvertent introduc-
       tion of large amounts of local anesthetic into the sys-
       temic circulation.
    3. The symptoms are proportional to the amount of
       local anesthetic introduced.
    4. They usually are referrable to:
       a. The central nervous system.
       b. The cardiovascular system.

    c. The respiratory system.

5. A *mild toxic reaction* may be characterized by nothing more than a feeling of warmth, light-headedness, dizziness and a feeling of being "high," a form of psychic instability.

6. It is easily managed by administration of oxygen, reassurance of the patient and the administration of a tranquilizer like promethazine (Phenergan), 10-25 mg., I.V.

7. More *severe* forms of toxic reactions will cause a more marked stimulation of the CNS leading to convulsions.
   a. Convulsions originally were managed by intravenous injection of short-acting barbiturates like sodium pentothal or sodium surital.
   b. This treatment is not necessary if the convulsions do not interfere with respiration.
   c. Administration of oxygen by face mask is all that may be needed.

8. CNS depression (general anesthesia) may occur after an initial CNS stimulation.
   a. The barbiturates can augment the CNS depressant action.
   b. As depression of the CNS increases, the local anesthetic starts to act as a general anesthetic and unconsciousness may ensue.
   c. Local anesthetics, in fact, have been employed as general anesthetics by intravenous administration.
   d. Since the distribution of local anesthetics depends upon the blood flow to any organ, it is not difficult to imagine that a massive dose will affect *respiratory* and *cardiovascular functions.*

9. Respiration may be diminished from action on the respiratory center and possible peripheral curarizing effects of the local anesthetic.

10. The local anesthetic can affect the membrane of the myocardial cell and depress cardiac output.

11. This effect on the myocardium has been utilized in the management of cardiac arrhythmias, e.g., lidocaine, procaine.

12. Peripherally, the local anesthetics may depress ganglia and smaller blood vessels causing dilatation and HYPOTENSION.

E. MANAGEMENT

1. Respiratory Failure.
   a. Establish a *patient airway* by inserting an intratracheal tube or by using an anesthesia face mask and assisting ventilation.

2. Cardiovascular Problems.
   a. Hypotension, which may be very severe, and occasionally bradycardia progressing to cardiac arrest, may be managed by administration of a vasopressor.
   b. It has been our practice to start an *I. V. drip* before administering any regional block, and it is *advisable* in the Emergency Service.
   c. It allows for administration of emergency resuscitative drugs, particularly in the treatment of cardiovascular problems.
   d. A 5% D/W or Ringer-lactate solution is preferable to normal saline.
   e. The brain metabolizes glucose primarily; its presence in the I.V. solution might be of great value.

3. Hypotension.
   a. Vasopressors should be limited to those that are mild, brief in action and easily controllable.
   b. A mild vasopressor for mild hypotension is either ephedrin, 5-15 mg., I.V., or desoxy-ephedrine, 5-10 mg., I.V.
   c. Should the hypotension be more severe, and an acute response needed, our choice is phenylephrine given either as a single dose, or as an I.V. drip.
      1) As a single dose, 1-2 mg. is diluted into 10 ml. of normal saline and given in small increments.
      2) The amount administered is dictated by the blood pressure response.

3) If the blood pressure is not maintained after a single dose of phenylephrine, a solution of 10-20 mg. in 250-500 ml. of 5% D/W is given as an I.V. drip. Again, the amount and rate of administration should be controlled by the blood pressure response.

F. HYPERSENSITIVITY

1. The response of the patient is very similar to a severe systemic reaction.
2. The main difference is that the amount of local anesthetic that had been administered before the reaction is quite small as compared to a true systemic reaction.
3. The *management* of this condition is very similar to that of a severe toxic reaction.

G. REACTION TO EPINEPHRINE

1. Epinephrine in small concentrations frequently is used to prolong the duration of the injection or block.
2. This is particularly true of *lidocaine* which tends to diffuse quickly and be absorbed rapidly.
3. This rapid absorption of the solution decreases the exposure time of the nerves and decreases anesthetic time.
4. The addition of epinephrine causes vasoconstriction and slows down absorption and diffusion of the drug.
5. However, absorption of the epinephrine itself, even though in minute amounts, can cause tachycardia, palpitation and occasionally "goose pimples."
6. Patients regard this as a reaction to the anesthetic.

H. FEAR

1. This reaction of an apprehensive patient may well account for most mild to severe toxic reactions to local anesthetics.
2. No matter how hard one tries to allay the patient's apprehension and explain the procedure to him, the fear of the needle or effects of the local anesthetic

such as numbness or paralysis may provoke severe apprehension.
3. Nausea and vomiting are probably the most common manifestations of this psychogenic reaction.
4. Serious complications such as hypotension, bradycardia or loss of consciousness may mimic a severe systemic toxic reaction.
5. For the milder forms, administration of a tranquilizer such as promethazine, 10-25 mg. I.V., is frequently sufficient.

IV. GENERAL ANESTHESIA

A. It is our feeling that every patient requiring a general anesthetic should:
1. Be taken to the Main Operating Suite.
2. Be admitted to the hospital.

B. Many aspects of general anesthesia in the adult emergency patient have been covered in the section on "Pediatric Anesthesia in the Emergency Service" and therefore will not be repeated.

CHAPTER 7

Prophylaxis of Tetanus and Rabies

STUART LEVIN, M.D.

I. PREVENTIVE TREATMENT OF TETANUS

A. GENERAL CONSIDERATIONS

1. Tetanus organisms cause very serious illness by toxin production even if confined to a circumscribed area of tissue damage.
2. Tetanus *prevention* is dependent:
   a. Primarily upon prophylactic *immunization.*
   b. Secondarily upon meticulous surgical care of wounds.
   c. The proper use of *human* tetanus antitoxin and tetanus toxoid.
3. The identification by smear and culture of this *anaerobic,* gram-positive, spore-forming bacillus is *not* essential for the use of prophylactic measures or the diagnosis and management of clinical tetanus.

B. IMMUNIZATION

1. Recent studies continue to corroborate that in patients with a history of adequate immunization consisting of 4-5 toxoid injections, there is no need for routine booster injections more often than every 10 years. Alum-precipitated (cloudy) tetanus toxoid is preferred, but fluid toxoid is acceptable.

C. TREATMENT OF PATIENTS WITHOUT GOOD EVIDENCE OF COMPLETE TOXOID IMMUNIZATION

1. The patients who have not had the basic series

should receive toxoid immunization with 0.5 ml. (cloudy) tetanus toxoid.

2. If the wound is a clean minor wound, then antitoxin is not necessary.

3. In moderately severe wounds, 250 units of tetanus immune globulin (human) should be given with a separate syringe and needle in a separate site.

4. There is *no reason* to use animal antitoxin for tetanus prophylaxis.

5. It is important to remember that tetanus can arise from *minor* injuries that do not receive good local care in patients that have been inadequately immunized.

D. INJURED PATIENTS WITH COMPLETE TETANUS TOXOID IMMUNIZATION

1. These patients *should not* receive toxoid boosters or human antitoxin if they have had a toxoid booster within the past 10 years *unless the presence of a very severe wound* significantly increases the possibility of tetanus.

2. In the case of a severely contaminated wound, *both* toxoid and human antitoxin should be given.

3. *Small penetrating wounds* are tetanus-prone.

4. The risk of inducing a serious allergic reaction to tetanus toxoid is greater than the likelihood of clinical tetanus developing in a patient who has had the basic series of immunization and a booster within 10 years.

5. Excluding the separate problems of tetanus neonatorum, the major groups developing tetanus include:

   a. Patients over 50 years of age.

   b. Narcotics addicts.

   c. Patients with chronic dermatologic conditions.

   d. These patients *in particular* should be immunized with the basic series if they have a negative past history of toxoid immunization.

   e. The basic series on these patients should consist of 2-3 monthly 0.5 ml. of tetanus toxoid, I.M., followed 6 months to a year later by a single 0.5 ml. booster.

E. *Meticulous care of the wound* is necessary in all injuries not only to prevent tetanus but also to prevent secondary infections.

F. Antibiotics *are not* substitutes for any of the above but should be given with a grossly contaminated wound that cannot be debrided adequately.
   1. *Dose:* 1.2 million units of procaine penicillin G, I.M., per day for 10 days or more is the drug of choice.
   2. Two grams in divided doses, of either erythromycin, tetracycline or lincomycin are reasonable substitutes. The last three drugs can be given orally, but are more dependable as I.V. injections.
   3. A patient with such a wound should be *admitted* to the hospital.

II. PREVENTIVE TREATMENT OF RABIES

A. GENERAL CONSIDERATIONS
   1. Rabies, caused by an RNA virus, is essentially a completely fatal illness in man.
   2. The prevention of rabies is different than the prophylactic regimens of any other infection in that active immunization usually is given *after* the possible infection has been introduced into the patients.
   3. Unfortunately, immunization alone is not yet a satisfactory method of prevention.

B. LOCAL CARE OF THE ANIMAL BITE
   1. The wound should be immediately and thoroughly flushed with a concentrated soap solution followed by 1% benzalkonium chloride. Forty to 70% ethanol (whiskey—86 proof) can be used if the patient is far from a physician or hospital.
   2. Flushing of the wound for 10-15 minutes with

catheters is strongly recommended. Nitric acid *should not* be used.
3. Debridement of damaged tissue *without* primary suturing is also very important.
4. It has been shown that wounds of the face can be treated by thorough, prolonged irrigation and meticulous closure with very fine sutures. However, bites that are likely to be rabid should *not* be closed.

C. VACCINATION AND ANTITOXIN THERAPY

1. The 1966 World Health Organization (WHO) recommendations on the use of rabies vaccine and rabies antitoxin should be followed (table).
2. However, the very *low* incidence of rabies in domestic cats and dogs in the United States and the relatively *high* risk of reactions to both rabbit brain vaccine (Semple) and rabies horse serum antitoxin have lead many authorities to re-evaluate these recommendations in the United States.

D. WILD ANIMAL BITES

1. The victims of unprovoked wild animal bites are often *undertreated* unless the animal is captured and found free of rabies.
2. In the past 10 years, most deaths from rabies in this country have occurred from wild animal bites with the major reservoirs being found in skunks, foxes, raccoons and bats.
3. The wild wolf, bobcat, badger and domestic cow, horse and goat should be considered potentially rabid if *unprovoked* bites are suffered.
   a. These patients should receive a basic series of:
      1) Rabies vaccine, either Duck Embryo Vaccine (DEV), or Semple nerve tissue vaccine (NTV), 1 ml. per day s.c. for 14 days.
      2) The very important boosters of 1 ml. at the 24th and 34th days.
      3) In addition, the patient *immediately,* or within *24 hours,* should have 40 units/kg. of rabies horse serum antitoxin.

        a) First, determine by the reaction to an intradermal or conjunctival 0.1 ml. dose of a 1-100 dilution of the serum that *acute hypersensitivity* is *not* present.

        b) Local administration of 50% of the total antitoxin dose around the wound, when possible, is felt to be useful.

        c) The rest of the dose is given I.M.

    4) In this author's opinion, Duck Embryo Vaccine has *not* proved sufficiently antigenic to warrant its use in serious bites by *definitely* rabid animals.

    5) The Semple nerve tissue vaccine (NTV) should be strongly considered unless reactions occur.

    6) In such a case, the full course of Duck Embryo Vaccine, including a 1 ml. booster on the 24th and 34th days, is given.

4. Most deaths from rabies probably are caused by:
   a. Rabies antitoxin never given.
   b. Rabies antitoxin given too long after the initial bite rather than within the recommended 24-hour period.

5. Experimentally, withholding antitoxin for more than 72 hours markedly diminishes its usefulness.

6. Patients allergic to eggs may have a reaction to DEV.

7. Bites from wild rodents (rats, mice, gophers, chipmunks, squirrels and hamsters) are *so much less likely* to inflict rabies that prophylaxis against rabies is not warranted unless the animal is proved rabid.
   a. Meticulous wound cleansing, however, *must* be performed.

E. DOMESTIC DOG AND CAT BITES

1. There are approximately 1/2 million dog bites per year in this country.

2. Meticulous, thorough irrigation and complete debridement are mandatory.

3. The risk of rabies from the bites of a dog or cat who has been immunized is so low (but still possible) that rabies prophylaxis should not be started unless the animal becomes rabid while under observation.

GUIDE FOR SPECIFIC POSTEXPOSURE TREATMENT*

Nature of Exposure	Status of Biting Animal (Whether Vaccinated or Not)		Recommended Treatment
	At time of exposure	During observation period of ten days	
I. No lesions; indirect contact.	(a) Rabid (?)+	(a) Healthy	(a) None
II. LICKS: (1) Unabraded skin (2) Abraded skin (3) Scratches (4) Unabraded or abraded mucosa	(a) Rabid,	(a) Healthy	(a) None, (start vaccine at first signs of rabies in the biting animal).
	(b) Healthy,	(b, c) Clinical signs of rabies or proved rabid (laboratory)	(b, c) Start vaccine immediately; stop treatment if animal is normal on fifth day after exposure.
	(c) Signs suggestive of rabies,		
	(d) Escaped, killed, or unknown.	(d) Not observed.	(d) Start vaccine immediately.
III. BITES: (1) Mild exposure	(a) Healthy	(a) Clinical signs of rabies or proved rabid (laboratory)	(a) Start vaccine at first signs of rabies in the biting animal.
	(b) Signs suggestive of rabies	(b) Healthy	(b) Start vaccine immediately; stop treatment if animal is normal on fifth day after exposure.

	(c) 1) Rabid, 2) Escaped, 3) Killed, or 4) Unknown	(c) ———	(c) Start serum immediately; then course of vaccine.
	(d) Wild: wolf, jackal, fox, bat, etc. See text.+	(d) ———	(d) Serum immediately; followed by a course of vaccine.
(2) Severe exposure a) face b) head c) finger d) neck or e) multiple bites.	(a) Healthy	(a) Clinical signs of rabies or proved rabid (laboratory)	(a) Serum immediately; start vaccine at first sign of rabies in biting animal.
	(b) Signs suggestive of rabies	(b) Healthy	(b) Serum immediately, followed by vaccine. Vaccine may be stopped if animal is normal on fifth day after exposure.
	(c) 1) Rabid, 2) Escaped, 3) Killed, or 4) Unknown	(c) ———	(c) Serum immediately, followed by vaccine.
	(d) Wild: wolf, jackal, pariah dog, fox, bat, etc. See text.+	(d) ———	(d) Serum immediately, followed by vaccine.

*Modified from the World Health Organization, Technical Report Series No. 321, Expert Committee on Rabies, Fifth Report, 1966.

+Editor's Note.

4. The occurrence of rabies in man from domestic dog or cat bites in the United States is almost unknown at this time.

5. A change in personality of an unprovoked, attacking domestic animal dictates *complete therapy,* both vaccine and antitoxin.

6. Bites by known hostile domestic animals should encourage *not* using either agent unless the animal is felt to be ill and potentially rabid.

7. Dog bites suffered by U.S. citizens in *other* countries must be considered potentially dangerous as the dog still remains an important vector in many other nations of the world.

F. SEMPLE (NTV) vs. DUCK EMBRYO VACCINE (DEV)

1. The tremendous acceptance of the Duck Embryo Vaccine (DEV) in this country unfortunately *does not* guarantee its efficacy.

2. There is definitely less hazard of inducing allergic encephalomyelitis when compared with the nerve tissue vaccine (Semple).

3. What is needed is an agent with the safety of DEV but with much more protective activity.

4. There are very few occasions when there is an indication for rabies vaccine without rabies antitoxin.

5. The hazard of serum sickness is less than the danger of a rabid animal bite.

6. The vast majority of patients with bites caused by rodents and domestic dogs and cats that do *not* receive antitoxin need not receive vaccine.

7. The patient who is bitten by an unprovoked wild animal that is not a rodent immediately should receive a *full course of antitoxin* and a *full course of vaccine* including the boosters at the 24th and 34th days.

8. Hopefully, in the future, a human rabies antitoxin and more antigenic and less encephalogenic vaccine will make the physician's decision more simple.

G. THE EMERGENCY SERVICE RECORD MUST SHOW

1. Whether the dog is known or stray.
2. Where it resides.
3. That the *police* have been notified.
4. That tetanus toxoid has been given unless the patient has received a booster within the last 5 years.
5. That a return appointment has been given.

H. ANTIBIOTICS

1. As with most surgical wounds, antibiotics are not a substitute for meticulous care of the wound.
2. The normal flora in the mouths of dogs and cats usually contains *pasturella multocida,* an important cause of infection.
3. *Pasturella multocida* is sensitive to penicillin, tetracycline and many other agents.
4. However, if the wound is not debrided and irrigated thoroughly, all antibiotics will fail in preventing infection.

CHAPTER 8

Thoracic Injuries

MILTON A. MEIER, M.D., FLOYD H. OKADA,
M.D. *and* DAVID M. LONG, JR., M.D.

I. GENERAL CONSIDERATIONS

A. Patients with injuries to the chest frequently are in critical condition and require rapid diagnosis and adequate treatment. Thoracotomy is needed in only 10-15% of cases of major thoracic trauma. The other 85-90% of cases need resuscitation procedures available in a well equipped Emergency Service.

B. The patient coming to the Emergency Service should be examined promptly to assess respiratory and circulatory functions. The examiner should:
   1. Listen to the mouth and nose of the patient.
   2. Watch the movements of the chest.
   3. Palpate the radial pulse.

C. Good air exchange reduces the possibility of impaired ventilatory function. If the air exchange is good, but the pulse is diminished, one should consider *cardiac tamponade* or a *massive hemothorax*.

D. If the exchange is poor despite vigorous respiratory efforts, look for:
   1. Airway obstruction.
   2. Open pneumothorax.
   3. Flail chest.

E. If the expired air is minimal, the chest wall does not move well and one hemithorax is prominent, a large pneumothorax or hemothorax may be present. The *neck* also should be examined for the position of the trachea, the presence of subcutaneous emphysema, distended neck veins and evidence of trauma.

II. INITIAL RESUSCITATION

See Chapter 1, "Cardiopulmonary Resuscitation."

A. Immediate artificial respiratory support must be started if:
   1. There is airway obstruction characterized by:
      a. Stridor.
      b. Diaphragmatic or intercostal retraction.
      c. Wheezing.
      d. Cyanosis.

B. A face mask with a non-rebreathing bag or mouth-to-mouth respiration are quick and effective ways to begin artificial respiration.

C. For *prolonged* respiratory resuscitation, direct endotracheal intubation with the use of a mechanical ventilator is more reliable.

D. In most cases, endotracheal intubation will provide an entirely adequate airway for hours or days. A tracheostomy, if required, can be done later on an elective basis.

E. An emergency tracheostomy is needed if there is complete or near complete *upper* airway obstruction.
   1. A cricothyroid "stab" and insertion of a tube can be lifesaving.
   2. The cricothyroid membrane can be palpated by feeling for the transverse indentation that is located below the thyroid cartilage.
   3. The trachea is opened and a tube is inserted to maintain patency.
   4. As soon as the condition of the patient permits, a lower tracheostomy should be performed. (See Chap. 2 and 3.)

III. DIAGNOSIS AND TREATMENT OF THORACIC TRAUMA

Trauma to the chest can be either blunt or penetrating and may result in injuries that range from a simple rib fracture to involvement of several intrathoracic organs with massive blood loss.

A. RIB FRACTURE

1. This is probably the most common of all thoracic injuries.
2. Pain may curtail respiration and may prevent an adequate cough.
3. Vital capacity is often reduced in elderly patients and may lead to atelectasis, pneumonia and death.
4. The patient who presents with a simple rib fracture, has the usual complaints of pain aggravated by coughing, deep breathing or changes in position.
5. A chest x-ray film, including rib detail, confirms the diagnosis and helps rule out the presence of an underlying pneumothorax or hemothorax.
6. **Treatment.**
   a. Pain is usually relieved with 60 mg. of codeine with 600 mg. of aspirin every 4 hours.
   b. The best means of managing severe pain from rib fractures is by intercostal block.
   c. Lidocaine (Xylocaine, 1% with epinephrine) is infiltrated around the intercostal nerves above and below the rib fracture.
   d. The site of injection is *posterior* to the fracture and the needle is introduced beneath the lower edge of the rib.
   e. Adhesive strapping is *not* recommended as it may restrict breathing.
   f. The patient should be admitted to the hospital if:
      1) The patient is elderly.
      2) There is underlying cardiorespiratory disease.
      3) There are significant associated injuries.
      4) Multiple fractures are present.

5) Significant subcutaneous emphysema is present.

g. Patients not admitted should return in 24 hours for re-examination and chest x-ray to rule out later complications and repeat intercostal nerve block if needed.

B. FLAIL CHEST

1. When several ribs and/or the sternum are fractured on both sides of the point of impact, an unstable or flail chest may result (Fig. 8-1).
2. The unsupported chest wall segment moves in a paradoxical fashion, collapsing during inspiration (negative intrapleural pressure) and expanding during expiration.
3. The major defect in the lung under the flail segment may be a progressive atelectasis.
4. Failure of the lungs to fill and empty synchronously causes the mediastinum to swing back and forth.

Fig. 8-1.—Flail chest.

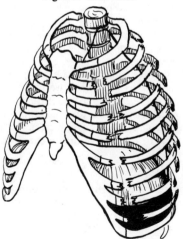

5. Possible major complications are:
    a. Oxygen *de*saturation due to the functional right-to-left shunt created by failure of ventilation.
    b. Impairment of effective coughing resulting in retention of secretions.
    c. Exhaustion due to the increased work of breathing.

6. **Treatment.**
    a. Stabilize the flail segment. This can be accomplished initially by firm, but gentle manual pressure or the use of sandbags. Another useful approach is to place the patient with the injured side down.
    b. Do *not use* clips or hooks passed around or through the flail segment.
    c. *Pain* should be relieved, preferably with intercostal block.
    d. If required, a face mask, with a respirator, should be used.
    e. In severe cases, *internal stabilization* is the best approach. Internal stabilization consists of insertion of an *airway* (endotracheal or nasotracheal) and *respiratory support* with a mechanical respirator.
    f. If it is apparent that respiratory support will have to be continued for days or weeks, a *tracheostomy* should be done.
    g. If there is an associated hemo-pneumothorax, chest tubes should be inserted.
    h. *Operative fixation* of fracture segments with internal wires and sutures is indicated if there are multiple fractures of the sternum, a large flail chest or bilateral injury to the thoracic cage.

C. PNEUMOTHORAX

1. Traumatic pneumothorax may follow blunt and penetrating injuries and can be associated with hemothorax. Air may gain access to the pleural space from several different sources.

2. The *amount* of air and whether it is under *tension must* be ascertained.
3. Small amounts of air may cause no symptoms and few physical signs. Usually, this type of pneumothorax is diagnosed only by a routine chest x-ray film (Fig. 8-2).
4. The *massive* accumulations will produce severe symptoms and signs:
   a. Dyspnea.
   b. Chest pain.
   c. Diminished breath sounds.
   d. Hyperresonance to percussion.
   e. A prominent but poorly moving hemithorax and cyanosis.
5. The most serious forms of pneumothorax are the *open* and *tension* types. The seriousness of open pneumothorax depends on the size of the opening.
   a. *Sucking chest wounds* are those in which the air is sucked into the pleural space by negative intrapleural pressure during inspiration.

Fig. 8-2.–Simple pneumothorax.

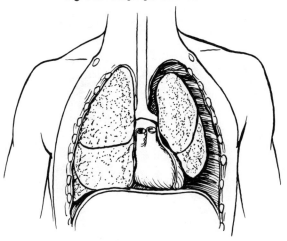

    b. Air moves in and out of the chest with a characteristic sound. The impairment to cardiorespiratory dynamics may be severe.

    c. If the opening is larger than the glottis, air will enter through the chest wall rather than through the trachea, a situation incompatible with life.

6. **Tension pneumothorax.**

    a. The leak of air into the pleural space is through an opening that acts as a one-way valve.

    b. The air enters the pleural cavity on inspiration but cannot escape during expiration.

    c. Pressure is built up, the lung collapses and the *mediastinum* swings to the opposite side with compression of the other lung (Fig. 8-3).

    d. Venous return to the heart is severely diminished.

    e. These patients have extreme dyspnea, severe cyanosis and signs of hypoxia.

Fig. 8-3.—Tension pneumothorax.

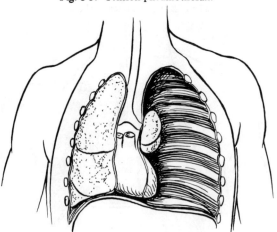

f. **Diagnosis.**
    1) Aspirate the chest with an 18-gauge needle
       and a syringe. The high intrapleural pressure
       will push the plunger of the syringe *outward.*

g. **Treatment.**
    1) *Simple pneumothorax:*
       a) With a small (10%) collapse.
       b) No increase in size.
       c) No dyspnea—*close* observation only is
          indicated.
       d) Repeat x-ray films should be made in 12-
          24 hours, or any time the symptoms
          worsen.
    2) *Large pneumothorax.*
       a) Tube thoracostomy and water-seal drain-
          age are indicated.
       b) Suction may be needed.
       c) Tube thoracostomy:
          i) The pleural cavity is entered in the
             sixth or seventh intercostal space at
             the midaxillary line (Fig. 8-4).
         ii) With local anesthesia, a small incision
             is made through the skin and muscles.
         iii) The *gloved finger* is then introduced
             into the wound to explore the pleural
             space. This collapses the lung further
             in partial pneumothorax and makes
             the insertion of the chest tube safer.
         iv) The tube can then be inserted using
             a curved hemostat.
          v) The tube is secured to the skin with
             sutures and *tape* and connected to a
             water-seal system.
         vi) A trocar should *not* be used; it is
             dangerous and only a small tube can
             be inserted through it.
    3) *Open pneumothorax.*
       a) The sucking wound must be immediately
          closed by any available means.
       b) This can be accomplished by the hand or
          a dressing with vaseline gauze.

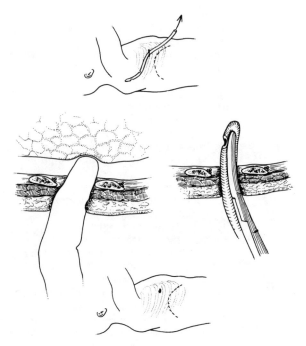

Fig. 8-4.–Chest tube insertion.

    c) *Tube drainage* of the thorax should be instituted as soon as possible.
    d) The patient is then taken to the operating room, if necessary, for definitive repair of the chest wall.

4) *Tension pneumothorax.*
    a) Air under tension must be removed *rapidly!*
    b) A large bore needle or any sharp instrument should be used to make a stab wound.

    c) This is performed safely through the *second* intercostal space in the midclavicular line.

    d) A chest tube with water-seal and suction are then inserted.

D. HEMOTHORAX

1. Hemothorax is an accumulation of blood in the pleural cavity and represents a very common finding in major chest trauma.

2. Lacerations of vessels of the chest wall, intrathoracic great vessels, or of the intrathoracic viscera (heart, lung and esophagus) may lead to:
   a. Hypovolemic shock.
   b. Compression of the lung.
   c. Hypoxemia and hypercapnia.

3. The symptoms will depend on the volume of blood in the pleural cavity and vary from minimal to severe shortness of breath and pain.

4. The physical *signs* of hemothorax are:
   a. Diminished breath sounds.
   b. Dullness to percussion over the involved hemithorax.
   c. Limitation of respiratory excursions.

5. A hemothorax of major proportions rarely is missed during physical examination. In lesser degrees of hemothorax, the diagnosis usually is made with an upright chest film.

6. **Treatment.**
   a. A minor hemothorax can be managed by thoracentesis alone.
   b. A major hemothorax is drained with a tube thoracostomy and connected to a water-seal and constant suction (-20 cm. of water).
   c. The blood is removed and the lung *must* be re-expanded.
   d. The chest tube should accurately indicate the rate of hemorrhage.
   e. Restoration of blood volume by fluid or blood

should begin immediately.
- f. Immediate thoracotomy is indicated in the following circumstances:
    1) Failure of the patient to respond fully to resuscitative measures and to maintain that response.
    2) Initial aspiration of more than 1,000 ml. of blood.
    3) Bleeding that continues at a rate of more than 250 ml. per hour or is steadily increasing.
    4) Inability to empty a large, clotted hemothorax and a shifted mediastinum.

E. LACERATION OF THE LUNG

1. Laceration of the lung results from penetrating trauma or from spicules of fractured ribs. *Pneumothorax* and *hemothorax* of varying degrees are always present and are treated as above.
2. The best method of controlling blood and air leaks from a lacerated lung is to *remove* all air and blood from the pleural space with a chest tube and to expand the lung completely.
3. Only the most severe lacerations need open thoracotomy and suturing or resection.

F. CONTUSION OF THE LUNG

See Chapter 9, "Emergencies of the Respiratory System."

1. An area of increased density in the chest x-ray film appears 12-72 hours after the injury. Areas of lung contusion are associated with hemorrhage; cavitation of the damaged area may occur later.
2. The term *wet lung* applies to severe lung contusion associated with voluminous tracheobronchial secretions, hemoptysis and pulmonary edema leading to hypoxia and hypercapnia.
3. Immediate endotracheal intubation to permit suctioning is indicated.
4. The patient should be placed on a mechanical

respirator with sufficient oxygen to maintain the arterial PO_2 above 60 mm. Hg.

G. TRACHEAL OR BRONCHIAL RUPTURE

1. Pneumomediastinum or pneumothorax usually is present.
2. Tension pneumothorax may occur.
3. Mediastinitis and compression of the trachea are the chief complications.
4. The presence of subcutaneous emphysema, especially in the neck, usually indicates a serious airway injury.
5. Bronchoscopy will establish the diagnosis.
6. Tracheostomy is used to control respiration, to remove secretions, and to prevent further leakage of air from the high intratracheal pressures that occur with coughing or a Valsalva maneuver.
7. A chest tube should be inserted if pneumothorax is present.
8. Operative repair of the tracheal or bronchial laceration is indicated as soon as possible after the patient is stable.

H. CHYLOTHORAX

1. Chylothorax is a rare complication of chest trauma and is due to injury of the thoracic duct.
2. The *diagnosis* is made when milky fluid is aspirated from the chest.
3. Accumulating chylous fluid is managed by chest tube drainage using continuous negative pressure.
4. Most chylous fistulae close spontaneously.
5. Some may require direct control of the leak by ligation of the thoracic duct just above the diaphragm through a right lower thoracotomy.

I. ESOPHAGEAL RUPTURE

1. Esophageal rupture may occur with either blunt or penetrating chest trauma.

2. The esophagus also may be *perforated* from *within* by a swallowed foreign body or during *esophagoscopy*.
3. It usually occurs at a point of constriction (the pharyngo-esophageal junction, the level of the aortic arch of the cardia).
4. The site of *rupture* is usually in the lower third just above the cardia and into the left chest. The mechanism of injury is *blunt trauma* or *forceful vomiting*.
5. *Symptoms*. The clinical picture is variable and depends upon the site of perforation or rupture and the degree of contamination.
    a. The patient complains of substernal pain due to spillage of esophageal content into the mediastinum; pain also may be felt in the epigastrum and in the neck.
    b. Severe mediastinitis, pneumomediastinum or left pneumohydrothorax may also be present.
    c. The *diagnosis* is confirmed by x-ray film studies performed with thin contrast media.
6. **Treatment.**
    a. The patient is given nothing by mouth.
    b. Intravenous fluids and broad spectrum antibiotics in large quantities are indicated.
    c. Repair of the defect usually should be done as soon as the diagnosis is made and if the condition of the patient permits.
    d. The pleural space should be drained *early* by tube thoracostomy.
    e. If there is a delay in diagnosis, both the mediastinum and the inevitable left pleural empyema should be drained at the site of rupture.
    f. If indicated, a diverting esophagocutaneous fistula is placed in the neck to prevent swallowing of saliva.
    g. A gastrostomy must be performed to aspirate gastric secretions and for feeding purposes.

J.   RUPTURE OF THE DIAPHRAGM

1. Rupture of the diaphragm often is seen after blunt trauma to either the chest or abdomen.
2. If the defect is large, bowel will herniate into the chest (Fig. 8-5). The tear is usually on the left.
3. Changes in respiratory physiology are much like those seen in flail chest.
4. With acute herniation, the first complaints are dyspnea and left chest pain which may be referred to the shoulder.
5. The *diagnosis* is made with the chest x-ray film. Do *not* confuse *herniated bowel* with *fluid!*
6. **Treatment.**—Operative reduction of the herniation and repair of the ruptured diaphragm are performed as soon as possible.

Fig. 8-5.—Diaphragmatic hernia.

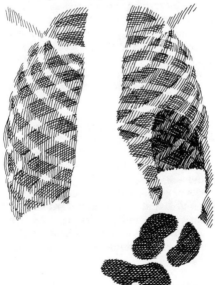

K. PENETRATING INJURIES TO THE HEART

1. Cardiac perforation may involve the walls of the cardiac chambers, the ventricular septum, or the valves.
2. Resultant septal defects, valvular insufficiency and infarction from injury to a coronary artery may occur.
3. Recurrent pericardial effusion or constrictive pericarditis may result.
4. Perforating cardiac injuries usually produce *hemopericardium* with *cardiac tamponade.* Some perforations of the heart seal spontaneously and do not require operative closure.

L. CARDIAC TAMPONADE

1. Cardiac tamponade occurs from an accumulation of blood in the pericardial sac.
2. Diastolic filling and stroke volume decline.
3. *Beck's triad* (falling arterial pressure, rising venous pressure and a quiet heart) is often present.
4. Severe shock out of proportion to the severity of the chest wound and the amount of blood lost, weighs heavily in favor of tamponade.
5. Another sign of cardiac tamponade is the "pulsus paradoxus," that is, weakening of the pulse during inspiration.
6. **Treatment.**
   a. Needle aspiration is the initial treatment and often is lifesaving (Fig. 8-6).
   b. Aspiration is performed with a 16- or 18-gauge short bevel needle attached to a 3-way stopcock and a 50-ml. syringe.
   c. The needle is inserted slightly to the left of the xyphoid and is pushed upward and to the left until blood can be aspirated. The depth of insertion usually is 3-4 cm. Unless there is great urgency, this should be done with ECG monitoring.
   d. After aspiration is performed the patient must be observed *continuously* in the operating room

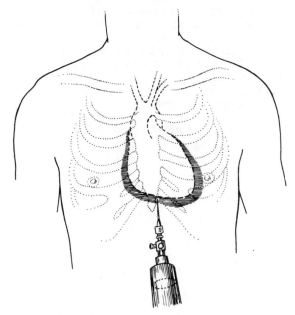

Fig. 8-6.–Needle aspiration of pericardial fluid.

or intensive care unit.

e. *Thoracotomy* is the definitive treatment for all patients with penetrating wounds of the heart with acute hemopericardium and tamponade.
1) All blood and clots must be evacuated.
2) The wounds of the heart should be closed.
3) A wide aperture is made in the pericardium to provide for drainage.

M. INJURIES TO THE AORTA AND GREAT VESSELS

1. *Penetrating* injuries to the aorta may result in cardiac tamponade or hemothorax, depending on whether the site of the vessel injury is intra- or extrapericardial.

2. *Nonpenetrating* injuries—the most common site of *rupture* is near the aortic isthmus just below the origin of the subclavian artery.
3. Such injuries usually are fatal immediately but a small number of these patients may survive long enough to reach the hospital.
4. **Treatment.**
    a. Immediate thoracotomy is indicated.
    b. The hemothorax is evacuated and the source of bleeding localized and controlled.

CHAPTER 9

Emergencies of the Respiratory System

SHELDON O. BURMAN, M.D., *and*
DECIO O. ELIAS, M.D.

The Emergency Service physician and the family practice physician frequently are called upon to diagnose and treat emergencies dealing with the respiratory system. Lifesaving measures may consist of emergency therapy only, but other cases must be followed by definitive therapy performed in the operating room or in an intensive care area. A significant number of these emergencies occur in the newborn infant.

A. NEONATAL RESPIRATORY DISTRESS

The cardinal signs of neonatal respiratory distress are: Tachypnea (respiratory rate over 40 per minute), dyspnea (marked by retractions or stridor) and cyanosis. Immediate adequate chest roentgenograms are needed to determine the possible presence of a surgically remediable congenital anomaly. The following conditions must be considered in the differential diagnosis:

1. *Choanal atresia.* – This is a membranous or bony occlusion of the posterior nares. The unilateral form may go undetected, but severe respiratory distress results from atresia of both posterior choanae because the newborn is incapable of sustained mouth breathing. Arching of the head and neck, severe suprasternal retraction on inspiration, a normal cry and inability to breathe while feeding are all characteristic. The *diagnosis* is confirmed by the inability

137

to pass a small catheter into the pharynx via either nostril.

   a. Emergency therapy—insertion of an oral airway which bypasses the point of obstruction.

   b. Definitive therapy—excision of atretic area usually via a transpalatal approach.

2. *Laryngeal webs and/or cysts.*—These are characterized by severe inspiratory obstruction with a normal cry. The lesion can be visualized with an infant laryngoscope. When widely incised, the cysts collapse and rarely recur. Webs are incised or excised under direct vision using a laryngoscope.

3. *Pneumothorax.*—This results from alveolar rupture during and following parturition. Overzealous artificial respiration is sometimes blamed, but pneumothorax frequently occurs without any efforts at resuscitation having been made. The tear may perforate the pleura producing a pneumothorax with ipsilateral lung collapse, contralateral shift of the mediastinum and severe respiratory distress. Air may remain interstitial in which case large amounts are trapped and the lung becomes extremely still and inelastic.

    Diagnosis is usually easy since, on a roentgenogram, a nubbin of collapsed lung is seen clustered at the hilum. Management of tension pneumothorax is most urgent and readily accomplished. Simple aspiration with a needle and syringe is followed by immediate improvement. A thoracotomy tube connected to underwater drainage, with or without negative pressure, allows air to escape while the lung expands and the tear seals. Direct suture of the leak is rarely necessary. Salvage may be impossible if the interstitial component is massive. Since the process is often *bilateral,* the unwary may insert one thoracotomy tube only to lose the baby because of the development of a contralateral lesion.

4. *Lobar emphysema.*—This is a rapidly ballooning, air-filled sac which is almost always confined to a single, usually upper, lobe, and is caused by incomplete bronchial obstruction that allows ingress of air dur-

ing inspiration but blocks egress during expiration. The obstruction is most often mural due to deficient cartilaginous support. It may be intraluminal due to intrinsic secretions, web, or vessel, or, rarely, extrinsic due to pressure from anomalous vessels or a ligamentum arteriosum.

Dyspnea, diminished excursion of the affected side with decreased breath sounds, hyperresonance and increasing cyanosis are characteristic. A radiolucent area in the lung fields with mediastinal shift, when seen on a roentgenogram, is suggestive of lobar emphysema or congenital lung cyst. The appearance of scattered lung markings in the area of radiolucency usually favors lobar emphysema rather than lung cyst or pneumothorax.

Emergency lobectomy is the treatment of choice. Needle aspiration may be done as an emergency measure as preparations are made for operation. Pneumothorax may result but is readily managed by a thoracotomy tube.

5. *Congenital lung cysts.* – These lesions may be generalized but are usually confined to a single lobe. They may balloon up rapidly and quickly compress the remaining pulmonary parenchyma. On the roentgenogram, a sharp outlining membrane usually can be seen and partition loculations may be present. *Immediate resection* is indicated. Catheter or needle decompression may be lifesaving, at the cost of a pneumothorax which itself is readily manageable.

6. *Congenital eventration of the diaphragm.* – In this condition one leaf of the diaphragm, usually the left, has defective musculature and ascends as a thin aponeurotic sheet high in the chest. All degrees of involvement exist from the asymptomatic to the rapidly fatal. *Diagnosis* is established by roentgenogram. Unlike phrenic nerve paralysis, synchronous motion is present in at least half of these patients. Emergency plication is done if respiratory embarrassment exists.

7. *Phrenic nerve paralysis.* – This is often associated with brachial paralysis. It is most commonly found in

large infants, on the right side and often related to dystocia. Infants with cyanosis, tachypnea, feeble cry, apneic spells and Erb's palsy should be fluoroscoped at once and paradoxic motion of the diaphragm will be seen. In the severely symptomatic infant, plication may be lifesaving.

8. *Diaphragmatic hernia.*—Displacement of abdominal viscera into the fetal chest is usually associated with diaphragmatic defects, usually posterior and left, through Bochdalek's foramen. Commonly the ipsilateral lung is hypoplastic, the mediastinum is shifted to the opposite side and the contralateral lung is somewhat compressed.

   a. *Diagnosis* is made by noting a scaphoid abdomen, tracheal deviation, ipsilateral decrease of breath sounds, apical heartbeat on the contralateral side and bowel sounds in the chest. The diagnosis is usually obvious on roentgenogram but if doubt exists a little contrast medium can be given.

   b. *Treatment* is indicated as soon as the diagnosis is made. Using an abdominal approach, the intestine is replaced within the abdomen and the defect closed. Frequently, associated malrotation and intrinsic gut webs are simultaneously corrected. Excessive efforts to inflate the hypoplastic lung are avoided; lung size and function gradually recover to normal or near normal.

9. *Hyaline membrane disease.*—The etiology of this syndrome is unknown. The lesion consists of an eosinophilic membrane lining alveolar ducts and alveoli. Resorptive atelectasis is prominent. Certain predisposing factors appear to be the male sex, prematurity, maternal hemorrhage and maternal diabetes mellitus. Neonates who have breathed entirely normally for 6-8 hours and then develop respiratory distress *do not* have hyaline membrane disease.

   a. Chest roentgenogram is the single, most useful diagnostic aid. The classic film shows diffuse, reticulogranular mottling throughout both lung fields, with the air-filled tracheobronchial tree in relief against the opacified perihilar area (air bronchogram). About half of all these patients will die regardless of therapy.

b. Those not desperately afflicted will respond to maintenance of body temperature, ventilatory assistance devices, correction of acidosis, the use of hypertonic glucose to spare protein catabolism and correction of anemia and hypovolemia. At the time of this writing, two pharmacologic agents appear promising: urokinase-activated human plasmin given intravenously and by aerosol, and estrogen, if given within the first 4 hours of life.

10. *Tracheo-esophageal fistula.* – In the most common form of this disorder, the proximal esophagus ends in a blind pouch at the level of the third or fourth thoracic vertebrae while the distal portion communicates with the trachea just above its bifurcation. The baby manifests excessive mucus which he cannot swallow and often aspirates. He chokes immediately upon the earliest attempt to feed him. The diagnosis is established when a catheter introduced through the nose fails to enter the stomach, although air in the gut is seen. Repair is extremely urgent and may be done in one or two stages.

B. LARYNGOTRACHEOBRONCHITIS (CROUP)

The onset of croup is frighteningly acute and occurs usually in children between the ages of 6 months and 3 years, with or without a preceding upper respiratory infection. The patients are febrile, toxic and provoke great concern.

The first symptoms are those of a barking cough associated with respiratory stridor and marked retraction, and the symptoms usually begin at night. The patient awakes with extreme anxiety and attempts violent inspiratory efforts. The child may rapidly develop severe dyspnea and, without adequate therapy, death may occur within a few minutes from complete occlusion of

the bronchial tree by thick viscid mucus or from a closure of the respiratory tract due to marked inflammatory edema of the larynx. There is usually a great
amount of thick tenacious mucus puddling at the lower
end of the trachea. The airway is narrowed by inflammatory reaction and edema of the mucosa and by spasm
of the bronchi.

Examination by the physician may cause complete
closure of the airway and should not be undertaken
without a tracheostomy set immediately available.
Many cases, including the most severe and fulminating,
are apparently associated with type B, *H. influenzae* infection. As soon as the case is diagnosed and until a culture directs otherwise, the child should receive antibiotics effective against H. influenzae.

Treatment:

1. Antibiotics.—In infants, for moderately severe infection, oral ampicillin in doses of 25-50 mg./kg. per
   24 hours in 4 divided doses is given. In more severe
   infections, 50-100 mg./kg. per 24 hours can be given
   orally or 50 mg./kg. per 24 hours in 4 divided doses
   can be given I.M. or I.V.

   In older children with moderately severe infection,
   50 mg./kg. per 24 hours in 4 divided doses is given
   orally; in more severe infections, 100 mg./kg. per 24
   hours I.M. or I.V. Children who are sensitive to penicillin should not receive ampicillin. If streptococci
   or pneumococci are cultured, this is treated with
   penicillin in doses of 20,000-50,000 units/kg. per
   day I.M. in 4 divided doses.

2. Maintenance of an adequate airway.
   a. In those instances where laryngeal spasm appears
      to predominate, the administration of syrup of
      ipecac may produce prompt relief of symptoms
      (*Caution:* **Syrup** of ipecac, *Not* Fluid Extract, is
      used). The dosage in infants up to 2 years is 1
      drop per month of age. In the older child, 2-5
      ml. may be given. These should be subemetic
      doses but vomiting occasionally may occur. Ob-
      serve carefully for aspiration. This dose may be

repeated after 1 hour if no vomiting has occurred and there is no relief of respiratory
symptoms.

b. Tracheostomy.—Tracheostomy is not a procedure to be undertaken lightly in infants and
children. It is sometimes followed by an unstable trachea which collapses easily following
withdrawal of the tracheostomy tube. However, when needed, it may be lifesaving. Considerable judgment and experience are necessary to
determine when tracheostomy is indicated. A
child upon whom a tracheostomy has been performed must be watched constantly because of
the small size of the tube which easily becomes
occluded by a plug of mucus. *Indications* for
tracheostomy are:
   1) A change in the child's color. (This does not
   necessarily mean cyanosis).
   2) A change in the child's behavior. A restless
   child who suddenly becomes quiet may be
   approaching the end of his energy reserves.
   3) Progressive elevation of pulse and a decrease
   in Po_2.

c. Oxygen and aerosol therapy: Oxygen administration is essential but dry oxygen dries and
thickens the mucus. It must be given in combination with aerosol therapy so that fine droplets
of normal saline or a mucolytic solution are inhaled through the open mouth. (Aerosol droplets are greatly decreased in number by nasal
breathing). The aerosol mist wets and soothes
the mucosa and thins the viscosity of the mucus,
allowing it to slide more freely. It frees the mucosal cilia which were held immobile by the dry-
ness and the thick mucus coating. The aerosol
mist may be given in the form of steam, but
when given cool it counteracts the inflammation
of the larynx. As a mucolytic agent, Acetyl-
cysteine (Mucomist) is most effective.

d. Hydration.—Children with croup should be kept

well hydrated. A fluid diet only should be given
and usually I.V. fluids should be started.

e. Sedation.—Most of these infants and children are
extremely anxious and anxiety increases the
spasm. Small amounts of mild sedatives frequently are useful. Chloral hydrate is the sedative of
choice and can be given by mouth or rectum.
The dose is 15 mg./kg. per 24 hours, not to exceed 1 g. daily. If given rectally, use a suppository or use cottonseed oil as a vehicle. It is important not to depress the respiratory center;
barbiturates are contraindicated.

f. Intermittent positive pressure breathing with
ventilator assistance requires cooperation and is
not tolerated except in older children.

g. Steroids.—There is no universal agreement regarding the efficacy of steroid therapy. It is
often used with the justification that it can do
little harm and may do some good.

C. ASPIRATION PNEUMONITIS

Aspiration pneumonitis usually is caused by inhalation of liquid or semi-solid vomitus. In the latter, death
can follow rapidly from acute asphyxia unless the obsta-
cle is dislodged. In the former type, highly acidic secretions enter the tracheobronchial tree. Bronchospasm
with severe wheezing, air hunger, anxiety, cyanosis,
tachypnea, tachycardia and hypotension may occur.
The condition simulates acute pulmonary edema, with
pink, frothy sputum, and bilateral rales and rhonchi.
The copious serosanguinous fluid impedes alveolar ventilation even though perfusion occurs, and the conse-
quent right-to-left shunting of blood in the lungs and the
decrease in pulmonary compliance add to the hypoxemia.

The principal early danger is death from hypoxia.
Early, the syndrome mimics congestive heart failure, pulmonary embolism, or amniotic fluid embolism; later it
resembles atelectasis and severe bronchopneumonia.
Chest roentgenography shows soft, diffuse, patchy

mottling with the right lower lobe involved most frequently and extensively.

Treatment.

1. Correction of the arterial desaturation secondary to physiologic right-to-left shunting by administering oxygen by mask or cannula in 40-100% concentrations, or, in more severe cases, by endotracheal intubation and positive pressure ventilation.
2. Gentle suctioning of the tracheobronchial tree to remove copious secretions.
3. Intratracheal instillation of 25 mg. of hydrocortisone in 10 ml. of normal saline.
4. If bronchospasm is severe, relieve with aminophylline 250 mg. I.V. in 500 ml. of 5% dextrose in water every 8 hours.
5. As soon as the diagnosis is made, give 100 mg. of hydrocortisone, then repeat every 8 hours for 72 hours and then 25 mg. every 6 hours for 2 additional days, with tapering thereafter.
6. Systemic antibiotics such as penicillin, streptomycin and methicillin.

D. WET LUNG SYNDROME

The boggy, edematous, stiff lung which characterizes this condition is usually the result of the lung being violently slammed against the chest wall. Agents usually responsible are steering wheel trauma, deceleration injuries and the concussion waves following explosions. Profuse interstitial petechial hemorrhages and massive transudation of fluid occur. The alveolar sacs and bronchi begin to fill with serous and serosanguinous secretions which form faster than they can be expectorated. Due to injury, pain and decreased lung compliance, the cough mechanism is impaired, compounding the problem. If unrelieved, hypoxia ensues and the patient becomes comatose and dies. Early in the syndrome the patient is apprehensive; respirations are rapid, shallow and often grunting. Dullness to percussion and decreased audible breath sounds are present. Coarse bilateral ronchi may be audible without aid of a stetho-scope. EARLY IN DEVELOPMENT OF WET LUNG, CHEST X-RAY FILM MAY SHOW LITTLE CHANGE IN LUNG FIELDS. SOON, HOWEVER, ATELEC-TASIS AND SUPERIMPOSED PNEUMONIA PRO-DUCE PULMONARY CONSOLIDATION.

Treatment.
1. Insertion of endotracheal tube or tracheostomy and ventilator-assisted respirations.
2. Antibiotics.
3. Mild analgesics. Do not depress the cough reflex.
4. If ribs are fractured, intercostal nerve block to re-lieve pain and improve coughing. (See Chap. 8, "Thoracic Injuries.")

E. RESPIRATORY BURNS

Fatal burns of the respiratory tract may occur with little or no external evidence. Pathologic changes are caused by inhalation of superheated air or toxic gases of combustion. Flame itself rarely penetrates beyond the upper respiratory tract. In the upper tract, edema may be so marked that obliteration and obstruction of the airway will occur. In such cases, tracheostomy must be done. Burns of the lower tract produce bronchial and bronchiolar epithelial desquamation plus severe edema and spasm. There is often a profuse outpouring of frothy fluid which may drown the patient.

Treatment.

The establishment and maintenance of a patent air-way is the key to treatment. Severe burns of the lower tract nearly always require that the patient be intubated or a tracheostomy be done and respirator-assisted ventilation be established. Antibiotics are useful. The mortality remains high, but less high than formerly. Patients with visible burns about the face and the mouth from fire or superheated air and who might otherwise be sent home after treatment in the emergency ward, should ordinarily be kept under observation for a period of several hours in case respiratory problems arise.

F. ATELECTASIS

Atlectasis is a state of incomplete expansion and airlessness of the lung due to failure of the air sacs to expand at birth (atelectasis of the newborn) or to the collapse of pulmonary alveoli. Collapse due to lung compression is usually readily reversible with the removal of the fluid, air or fibrous tissue (decortication) from the pleural space, provided the underlying lung is expandable. Atelectasis distal to endobronchial obstruction, such as bronchogenic neoplasm, may provide a helpful clue to diagnosis.

Atelectasis is one of the most common causes of postoperative morbidity and if uncorrected may produce arterial desaturation (physiologic right-to-left shunt), lung abscess or bronchiectasis. In children, aspiration of foreign bodies and cystic fibrosis of the pancreas associated with inspissated mucus plugs are common causes. In non-postoperative adults, endobronchial tumors, stenosing inflammatory diseases, aspiration of foreign material and chronic bronchopulmonary disease such as bronchitis, emphysema and asthma are the usual predisposing causes. In postoperative patients, alkalosis with respiratory paralysis, oversedation, overmedication with muscle relaxants, old age and debility, pain and apprehension and chronic bronchopulmonary disease are the usual precursors.

The clinical picture varies with the acuteness of onset and the extent of involvement. Patients with complete collapse of a lung which has been gradual in onset may be asymptomatic even with exercise. Sudden segmental collapse may produce fever, tachycardia, tachypnea and anxiety. Auscultation reveals crepitant rales and hyperresonance. The diagnosis is confirmed on the chest roentgenogram.

Treatment.

Treatment involves removal of the predisposing cause. Blood, fluid, air, fibrous tissue or foreign bodies must be removed from the pleural space. The tracheobronchial tree must be cleansed of obstructing material. Sitting the patient upright, encouraging him to cough, early ambulation, judicious administration of pain medication and nasotracheal aspiration by catheter are all useful in the postoperative period. If prompt improvement does not result, bronchoscopy may be both diagnostic and therapeutic and should be resorted to promptly. If secretions are copious and tenacious, endotracheal intubation or tracheostomy may be necessary.

G. WHEEZING

1. Wheezing indicates obstruction, but "all that wheezes is not asthma." The following are the most common causes of wheezing:
   a. Asthma.
   b. Chronic bronchitis or bronchiectasis.
   c. Heart failure.
   d. Aspiration of a foreign body.
   e. Stricture.
   f. Croup.
   g. Poisoning with cholinergic drugs or insecticides.
   h. Carcinoid tumors which elaborate serotonin.
   i. Chemical pneumonias such as silo-filler's disease.
2. *Differential diagnosis of wheezing.*

   When obstruction is situated in the larynx or trachea, the wheezing is generally higher pitched and may occur in inspiration or else the wheezes are at least as loud in inspiration as in expiration. This is characteristic of stridor, in contradistinction to the wheezing that originates in the bronchi. In asthma, the wheezing is caused by spasm of the smaller bronchi and is predominantly expiratory with prolongation of the expiratory phase of respiration. Special attention should be paid to the single-pitched wheezing rale which is usually due to obstruction of a larger bronchus. In infants and children it is usually on the right side *and is usually due to aspiration of a* **Foreign Object.** In adults it may be due to a plug of mucus but, more important, a neoplasm, stricture, foreign body or calcified, tuberculous extrinsic node. The wheezing of bronchial spasm may often be differentiated from that caused by thick mucoid secretion by observing the effects of coughing. Wheezing due to bronchial spasm is usually accentuated by coughing while wheezing due to secretions is usually diminished or abolished.

3. *"Cardiac asthma"* is an expression of incipient pulmonary edema, involving the interstitial tissue rather than the alveoli. The wheezing is in fact largely due to bronchial spasm as in allergic asthma, but the spasm is probably due to the edema of the tissue around the bronchi and blood vessels. The differentiation between an attack of pulmonary edema and bronchial asthma may be difficult since primary allergic asthma of long duration may eventuate into cor pulmonale. If the patient produces thin, frothy, bloody fluid, containing heart failure cells, the diagnosis is quite evident. Cardiomegaly, known history of valvar or coronary artery disease or myocardial infarction, and evidence of increased venous pressure suggest congestive failure rather than asthma. In bronchial asthma, an allergic history and exposure to known incitants help establish the diagnosis. Roentgenograms are usually very helpful. In asthma the lungs are perfectly clear, whereas in pulmonary edema they may show extensive clouding or short parallel lines at the lung bases (Kerley's lines).

4. *Chronic bronchitis, emphysema, bronchiectasis* or any condition where secretions are excessive or inadequately cleared may produce wheezing. In infants and children, aspiration of foreign bodies must be thought of first, especially in the absence of previous history of asthma.

    Croup (see above) has a rather typical nocturnal onset. If the etiology is obscure, bronchoscopy may be helpful. Bronchography will reveal a more distal obstruction where the bronchoscope cannot reach.

5. **Treatment.**
    a. *Bronchial asthma.*—Mild attacks are readily relieved by inhalation of 50-150 mg. of nebulized isoproterenol. With a rapidly developing severe

paroxysm, 0.3-1.0 ml. of 1:1000 epinephrine
should be injected s.c. and can be repeated no
oftener than once every 30 minutes. Tachyphy-
laxis is common. Aminophylline I.V. or rectally
is very effective and is given in 0.5 Gm. doses
slowly I.V. in 50 ml. of 5% glucose, or as a rectal
suppository. If epinephrine and aminophylline
are not adequate, 100-300 mg. of hydrocortisone may be given I.V. Once begun, steroids
should be continued until improvement occurs,
then tapered off.

b. For *cardiac asthma,* the usual therapeutic modes
for treatment of congestive heart failure will usually suffice.

c. *Foreign bodies* in infants and small children can
sometimes be dislodged manually. Failing this,
invert the patient and strike him sharply between
the scapulae. Success may occur only with repeated efforts. If airway obstruction is complete
and the patient becomes hypoxic, the object may
become dislodged as flaccidity of the patient ensues. Failure to extract a foreign object from the
pharynx, larynx or proximal trachea should be
followed by emergency tracheostomy. Endo-
scopic removal of a more distal object often requires special experience and equipment. In
children and some adults, general anesthesia is
necessary. Success is most often obtained by
passing an instrument through the bronchoscope
distal to the object and drawing it proximally until it can be grasped.

d. In *chronic bronchitis, bronchiectasis and emphysema,* cure of wheezing depends upon removal
of the copious, usually tenacious secretions. Patients with a cough reflex and sufficient vigor
will respond to liquefaction of secretions and
bronchodilators. High humidity atmosphere,
aerosol inhalations of water or dilute acetyl-
cysteine (Mucomist) and aminophylline by I.V.
drip or rectal suppository usually suffice. Dilute

nebulized isoproterenol will aid more refractory cases. Where the cough reflex is weak and body vigor is insufficient, secretions must be mechanically removed by catheter aspiration of the tracheobronchial tree or, rarely, by bronchoscopy. If secretions reaccumulate rapidly, a temporary tracheostomy may be necessary.

H. HEMOPTYSIS

Bleeding from the respiratory tract nearly always produces severe apprehension and prompts early medical consultation. It is first necessary to determine that the blood is not coming from the G.I. tract or nasopharynx. Blood from the gums or nasopharynx is usually bright red and not frothy. Blood from the gut is usually brownish-red. Blood from the lungs is usually bright red, frothy, mixed with phlegm and is associated with coughing or a "lump in the throat." Probably the single most common cause of hemoptysis is chronic bronchitis. Other common causes are pneumonia, tuberculosis, bronchiectasis, lung abscess, neoplasms, chronic passive congestion and pulmonary emboli. Emphysema rarely causes hemoptysis. Hemoptysis is particularly prevalent in pulmonary vascular congestion secondary to mitral stenosis. Coagulopathies, leukemia, pulmonary arteriovenous fistulas and anticoagulant therapy are other less common predisposing factors.

Since the discovery of antituberculous drugs, exsanguinating hemoptysis has become rare and emergency treatment is rarely necessary except perhaps to neutralize excessive anticoagulation. When bleeding is severe, the diagnosis can usually be elicited by a careful history and physical examination and chest roentgenogram. When bilateral lesions are present or the chest x-ray film is unremarkable, emergency bronchoscopy should be done during active bleeding to ascertain, if nothing else, which side the blood is coming from in case severe bleeding should necessitate emergency lung resection.

I. ACUTE RESPIRATORY FAILURE

The clinical features of acute respiratory failure may be obvious and dramatic or so subtle and insidious that the gravity of an imminent emergency is disregarded. The gasping, desperate patient struggling for breath evokes a prompt response, but the somnolent, noncomplaining patient with barely perceptible respirations and a silent chest may be in equally desperate straits. The signs of acute respiratory failure are those produced by hypoxia and hypercapnea upon the circulatory and central nervous system. These include headache, sweating, confusion and other mental aberrations, hypotension, tachycardia, cyanosis and unconsciousness. Arterial blood gas studies show elevation in Pco_2 and decrease in Po_2. The most common chronic causes are bronchitis and obstructive emphysema. The acute causes are any factors responsible for airway obstruction at any level.

The patient with chronic disease usually has overproduction of viscid tenacious sputum. Cough is often ineffective due to chronic infection or from loss of ciliary function due to cigarette smoking. Infection, excessive and abnormally thick sputum, bronchospasm, and alteration of blood gases are potentially reversible and in exhausted, debilitated patients the work of breathing can be diminished.

1. *Care of the airway.* The first principle is avoidance of irritants such as cigarette smoke and air pollutants. Next, clear the airway of secretions. Nasotracheal aspiration alternating frequently with periods of rest and oxygenation will usually accomplish this. Overzealous suctioning of a hypoxic patient may provoke a fatal arrythmia. Measures to liquify the sputum should be used. Systemic hydration is essential.

Warm, moist air inhaled orally is probably the single most effective agent in reducing sputum viscosity. Pharmacologic agents include oral potassium iodide, inhaled detergents such as Alevaire, and mucolytic agents such as acetyl cysteine (Mucomist). Postural drainage is helpful. For initial clearing of

obstructive secretions, therapeutic bronchoscopy
may be necessary. If these measures do not afford
prompt and prolonged relief, endotracheal intubation may be required. Indications are (1) inability
to control secretions by other methods, (2) continued rise in Po_2 and/or fall in Po_2, and (3) clinical
deterioration.

2. *Relief of bronchospasm.* Often, removal of secretions or control of incipient of actual heart failure
will suffice to correct bronchospasm. Aminophylline,
0.5 Gm. in a slow I.V. drip or by rectal suppository
is usually helpful. Inhaled isoproterenol 1:200 concentration by powered nebulizer, and systemic corticosteroids are likewise helpful. (See section on
Bronchial Asthma.) After initial relief, bronchial di-
lators and corticosteroids should be administered on
a consistent schedule.

3. *Oxygenation.* All patients in acute respiratory distress should receive oxygen therapy. The method
and percentage of oxygen administration will depend
on the patient's response. A nasal clip or nasopharyngeal catheter carrying 30-100% oxygen may suffice.
If the patient will tolerate it, a tight fitting mask is
more efficient.

In the acutely ill or exhausted patient, assisted
ventilation by some type of mechanical ventilator is
essential. Mechanical respirators are either volume-
regulated or pressure-regulated, depending upon the
factor responsible for terminating the inspiratory
phase. Volume-regulation is generally more effective
in patients depending for survival upon the machine.
The Bennett and Bird machines are examples of the
pressure-regulated type and can be used both to
assist and control respirations. They do not compensate for increased airway resistance and, being
pressure-sensitive, the inspiratory phase will become
shorter and shorter if secretions in the respiratory
tree accumulate. Furthermore, any airway leak will
prevent proper function.

Cylinder-and-piston respirators such as the Emerson, Morch, and Bennett are volume-limited. They can overcome tremendous airway resistance and can ventilate a very noncompliant chest. Cuffed tracheal tubes must not be used since air must escape through the larynx to avoid pressure build-up. These machines are very useful in those patients who require prolonged assistance.

In chronically hypoxic and hypercapneic patients, ventilator assistance may produce apnea due to the removal of the CNS respiratory stimulus. In such patients oxygen administration must be carefully controlled and abnormal Pco_2 and Po_2 values should be altered gradually.

4. *Infection.* In acute respiratory failure, infection is almost always present and sputum smears and cultures are mandatory. Broad spectrum antibiotics should be started at once and the regimen altered as dictated by subsequent results of the cultures and smears.

5. *Electrolyte replacement.* Excessive potassium and chloride loss is often seen in patients with acute respiratory failure. As they recover, hypokalemic and hypochloremic alkalosis becomes increasingly manifest and potassium chloride should be supplied if renal function is adequate.

6. *Cor pulmonale.* Chronic hypoxemia and acidosis produces pulmonary vasoconstriction which, by taxing the right side of the heart, can produce congestive failure. Cardiac glycosides, diuretics—the usual therapeutic regimen—are usually indicated.

CHAPTER 10

Acute Abdominal Emergencies

WILLIAM H. REQUARTH, M.D.

I. INTRODUCTION

A. It is well known that the chance to cure many acute abdominal emergencies lies in the narrow space of a few hours. It is essential that the physicians make the right decision as to whether an early operation is necessary.

B. Accuracy of diagnosis is best achieved by *exclusion* of groups of diseases in order to narrow the possibilities. For example, it is helpful during the initial examination to classify the cause of acute pain as either:
   1. A nonsurgical disease.
   2. Intestinal obstruction.
   3. An inflammatory disease, such as cholecystitis or appendicitis.

   The Emergency Service physician will also be called on to evaluate patients who have suffered trauma to the abdomen, and this will be considered apart from the so-called "acute abdomen."

C. The most diagnostic feature of *nonsurgical* disease is the *inconsistency* of the physical findings.
   1. Pain, even though severe, shifts from place to place.
   2. There is vomiting at the onset and possibly at intervals later, but during the free periods the patient not only does not vomit, but may take food by mouth.
   3. Anorexia is not persistent.
   4. The tenderness of nonsurgical lesions is usually mild; but—*more important*—it is *shifting* and *inconsistent*.
   5. It usually is safe to observe for a few hours a patient who presents a picture of diffuse pain and inconsistent, shifting tenderness.

6. The fact that bowel sounds are often normal in quality and frequency helps to corroborate the suspicion that no surgical disease exists.

D. Persistent tenderness, no matter how slight, is very significant, especially if it becomes *localized*.
1. If doubt exists as to the diagnosis, it is best to *delay* the decision to avoid the possibility of operating for a nonsurgical disease. It may not only be unnecessary, but may be contraindicated, as, for example, in coronary occlusion.
2. The pain of *coronary occlusion* is often in the upper abdomen and frequently substernal.
3. There may be a history of hypertension, previous disease or history of similar pain in the past caused by exertion.
4. The pain typically radiates to both shoulders or down the left arm.
5. Although the pain may be quite severe with myocardial infarction, the patient moves about the bed quite freely, in contrast to a patient with inflammatory disease, who is more likely to hold himself quite still.
6. Tenderness and rigidity of the upper abdomen is inconsistent, shifts about and usually is minimal.

II. INTESTINAL OBSTRUCTION

A. Mechanical obstruction of the bowel is a common cause of acute abdominal pain and should be diagnosed or excluded *early* by the physician.
1. The diagnosis of obstruction is not difficult and once it is established, it is important to *determine as early as possible* whether the *small* or *large* bowel is primarily involved.
2. From almost every clinical standpoint, obstructions of the small and large bowel are *two different diseases,* and the sooner one accepts this concept, the easier will be clinical management of these cases.

B. The *diagnosis* of obstruction cannot be made by any *single* group of symptoms.

1. Nearly all patients at some time during the course of obstruction have pain, vomiting, distention, obstipation and abnormal x-ray findings.
2. Distention and obstipation occur most consistently; yet neither is diagnostic.
3. Pain and vomiting are more prominent in *small bowel* obstructions and may be absent in obstructions of the large bowel.
4. Obstructive pain is typically *cramping,* occasionally simulated in such nonsurgical diseases as enteritis.
5. The pain of intestinal obstruction starts without warning, is frequently followed by vomiting, tends to build up to a peak of severity and then suddenly subsides.
   a. The next seizure follows in 5-15 minutes.
   b. Such rhythmic periodicity is characteristic of obstructive pain and differentiates it from cramping of minor intestinal disturbances.
6. The vomiting varies somewhat with the level of the obstruction, being frequent and abundant with *high* obstructions and occasionally absent in colon obstructions because the ileocecal valve prevents regurgitation.
7. Although absence of bowel movement is a natural sequence to mechanical block, a preliminary period of diarrhea may occur as the obstruction becomes complete.
8. Stool may be passed for as long as 24 hours after the onset while the colon is being evacuated.

C. *Distention* is *invariably* present unless the obstruction is quite high.
   1. Ordinarily, the distention begins in the lower abdomen and progresses upward as more and more loops become distended.

D. A characteristic finding in intestinal obstruction is the frequent presence of an obstructive type of *bowel sound* which results when intestinal contents are squirted through a narrow lumen. The sound may be followed by relief from pain, and this identifies that pain as an obstructive paroxysm.

E. The plain x-ray film of the abdomen made without the use of opaque media supplies important information for the diagnosis of obstruction and especially for differentiation between that of the small bowel and large bowel.
   1. Films should be made in both the supine and upright positions and should include the diaphragm and the lowest part of the pelvis.
   2. The film should be made *before* gastric suction or enemas are started because the *absence* of air in the stomach is strong evidence against the diagnosis of obstruction *unless* the patient has recently vomited.
   3. Cleansing enemas may not only produce confusing *fluid levels* in the colon but put gas in the *rectum,* which is *rarely present* in complete mechanical obstruction.

F. Normally, stasis does not occur in the gastrointestinal tract and air is seen *only* in the stomach or colon, and then only in small amounts.
   1. The appearance of even a small amount of gas in the *small* intestine indicates that there is some obstruction in the normal intestinal flow, either mechanical or adynamic.
   2. It is rare for gas *not* to be present in the colon.
   3. In the presence of a colonic obstruction, the amount of gas in the colon is greatly increased.

G. Gas in the intestinal tract produces typical patterns which identify the bowel as either *small* intestine or *colon.*
   1. Gas patterns are not always seen if only a supine film is made because the damming up of fluid proximal to the obstruction obliterates the gas pattern.
   2. The upright film will show multiple horizontal fluid levels which prove the existence of stasis.

H. It is most important to differentiate mechanical obstruction from *adynamic ileus,* with which it is often confused and for which operation is definitely contraindicated.
   1. Adynamic ileus follows a great variety of diseases, such as peritonitis, excessive trauma during surgery, injury to intra-abdominal organs and in a reflex manner after certain medical diseases.

   2. *Pain* is often absent except in postoperative ileus.
   3. The distention of the abdomen and the bowel is not progressive as in mechanical obstruction.
   4. Bowel sounds are characteristically absent.
   5. The plain x-ray film of the abdomen (Fig. 10-1) shows distended loops of both large and small bowel with *multiple fluid levels.*
   6. In mechanical obstruction, either the small or the large bowel is predominantly involved, depending on the level of the obstruction.

I. The differentiation between large and small bowel obstruction usually is not difficult. The typical *small* bowel obstruction is seen in the young or middle-aged patient.
   1. The patient usually has a *scar on the abdomen.*
   2. The obstruction is *sudden* in onset without antecedent symptoms and is accompanied by *severe pain* and *persistent vomiting.*

Fig. 10-1.—Adynamic ileus. Man, aged 58, fell on drawbar of tractor and suffered severe contusion of abdomen. Ileus suspected because of gas in both large and small bowels and only moderate distention of bowel.

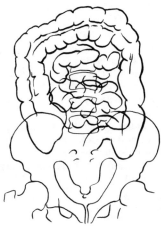

3. Conversely, *large bowel obstructions,* because they are usually caused by carcinoma, are seen mostly in older persons.

4. The history is one of chronic constipation, slowly progressing to *obstipation* with episodes of pain and bloating and frequently the passage of blood.

5. *Vomiting* is often minimal or absent.

6. X-ray interpretation of plain films of the abdomen is again a most valuable diagnostic procedure.

7. *Mechanical* obstruction primarily involves *either* the small intestine or the colon; gas appears in one or the other but rarely in both.

8. The characteristic small bowel pattern is that of distended bowel marked by thin feathery lines, the valvulae conniventes (Fig. 10-2).

9. The pattern of colon obstruction is one which outlines the *haustra* of the colon as large segmented collections of gas (Fig. 10-3).

10. One should not hesitate to use the *barium enema* freely for proper interpretation of plain films of the abdomen.

11. In the case of colon obstruction, the barium enema is *diagnostic* and seldom should be omitted.

J. *Recognition of strangulation* is not easy at any time, but the problem is simplified if the surgeon knows which lesions can produce it and is on the alert for them.

1. Strangulation rarely occurs in a large bowel obstruction except in volvulus.

2. Most colon obstructions are caused by a *neoplasm.*

3. In the few that are caused by *volvulus,* strangulation is a definite possibility, but the clinical picture is usually obvious.

4. If the patient is known to have large bowel obstruction and volvulus is ruled out, the possibility of *strangulation* is eliminated.

5. In contrast, *strangulation* is a constant hazard in all *small* bowel obstructions.

6. The most significant clinical finding is abdominal tenderness of varying intensity, usually associated with rebound tenderness.

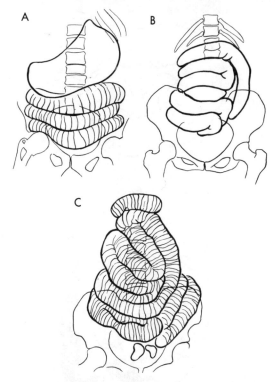

Fig. 10-2.—Mechanical small-bowel obstruction. **A,** bowel caught in implant of carcinoma. Valvulae conniventes identify pattern as small bowel. Gastrectasis present. **B,** valvulae conniventes not seen, but "ladder formation" identifies gas pattern as small-bowel obstruction (due to postoperative adhesion). **C,** advanced obstruction indicated by oblique position of loops in obstruction secondary to adhesion. The almost complete absence of air in the large bowel is characteristic of complete small-bowel obstruction.

7. The obstructive pain which at first is periodic tends to become constant and of great severity.

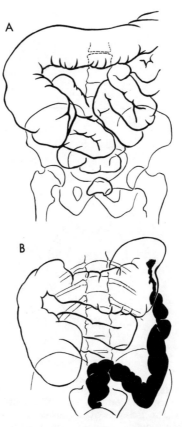

Fig. 10-3.—Large-bowel obstruction. **A,** diagram from plain film of abdomen showing distended cecum and transverse colon. The distended small bowel indicates incompetence of ileocecal valve and advanced obstruction. **B,** a suspected colon obstruction should be confirmed by barium enema.

III. ACUTE INFLAMMATORY DISEASE

A. The following applies to:
1. Appendicitis.
2. Cholecystitis.
3. Diverticulitis.
4. Pelvic inflammatory disease.

B. The *exact time of onset* must be determined since ensuing changes in the pathology and symptoms and signs correlate well.
1. If the patient is seen early, 2-4 hours after onset, it usually is safe to wait for unequivocal signs and symptoms; however, the patient must be examined at least *hourly* by the *same (experienced)* surgeon.
2. If acute symptoms develop suddenly, suggesting impending perforation or strangulation, the patient must have an *immediate* laparotomy.
3. There can be *no* excuse for delay unless the patient is extremely ill from quickly correctible causes, i.e., dehydration, anemia, cardiac or pulmonary decompensation—these must be corrected *rapidly* so that an intra-abdominal catastrophe can be prevented.
4. This is the *surgeon's* responsibility—he must take charge completely. No delay is allowed.
5. On an average, a decision must be made 15-24 hours after onset—but in many adults, and especially in children, symptoms may worsen very rapidly.
6. As a rule, if the patient appears 2 or 3 days after the onset of symptoms, peritonitis with distention and ileus or an inflammatory mass will be present.
7. Advanced disease can be present in the gallbladder with relatively minimal clinical findings.

C. The pain of inflammatory disease frequently begins slowly, *away* from the involved organ, and later tends to shift and localize over the organ.
1. It is often described as cramping, but it does not have the definite periodic seizure similar to the seizures of obstruction—and more important is the fact that

some pain persists at all times, even between the periods of intense pain.

2. The pain of intestinal obstruction is intermittent rather than remittent, i.e., between episodes, the patient is free from pain.

3. A particular feature of an acute inflammatory lesion is the production of pain when the patient walks, moves about or is jarred.

4. Other findings are elevation of rectal temperature and leukocytosis.

5. Abdominal pain which is severe enough to demand narcosis is likely to be "surgical" in origin, frequently requiring operative intervention.

D. LOWER ABDOMINAL PAIN

1. The key to diagnosis of lower abdominal pain, and possibly to all acute diseases of the abdomen, is a thorough knowledge of appendicitis.

2. Appendicitis accounts for about *half* of all acute abdominal conditions and ranks first in frequency and importance.

   a. Pathognomonic of acute appendicitis is generalized abdominal pain which later localizes to the right lower quadrant.

   b. Vomiting may be absent, but anorexia is always present.

   c. *Hunger* in a patient with abdominal pain speaks strongly *against* the diagnosis of appendicitis.

   d. The presence of localized abdominal tenderness on deep, careful palpation, no matter how slight, must be *evaluated with great care.*

   e. Localized tenderness in a patient who still has an appendix must be treated as appendicitis until ruled out.

   f. A low-lying appendix produces lower abdominal pain and tenderness which does not localize well, but usually can be diagnosed by rectal tenderness on the right.

   g. If the diagnosis is uncertain, any patient who has abdominal pain with localized tenderness in

the right lower quadrant usually will require
laparotomy.

3. The pain of *pelvic inflammatory disease* starts in the
lower abdomen, is quite persistent and may be severe; yet, the patient does not appear particularly ill.

   a. Because the gastrointestinal tract is not involved,
   it is not unusual for the patient to take food regularly.

   b. Tenderness is usually bilateral, although unfortunately, it frequently is localized in the right
   lower quadrant.

   c. Adnexal tenderness and—*most important*—ex-
   cruciating pain on movement of the cervix is of
   considerable diagnostic significance.

   d. The gonococcus may be obtained on smears
   from the cervix or Skene's or Bartholin's glands
   (see Part I, 4).

4. *Acute diverticulitis* produces symptoms similar to
those of appendicitis except that the findings are
localized to the *left* abdomen, are more often seen
in the older patient, and there may be previous x-ray
evidence of diverticulosis.

E. DIFFERENTIAL DIAGNOSIS

1. *Upper abdominal pain* is somewhat different in pattern from that of lower abdominal pain.

2. The *biliary tract* must receive first consideration because of the frequency of biliary disease and its
ability to mimic other acute upper abdominal diseases.

   a. Gallbladder pain characteristically is in the right
   upper quadrant or epigastrium with radiation
   through to the interscapular region and shoulder.

   b. Pain in *other* parts of the abdomen of more than
   a few hours' duration usually *does not* arise from
   the biliary tract.

   c. Tenderness over the gallbladder is *frequent,* and
   occasionally there is significant rise in the quan-
   titative serum bilirubin, even though there is no
   stone in the common bile duct.

3. **Perforated peptic ulcer.**
   a. If the clinical signs are suggestive, upright and left lateral decubitus x-ray films are taken to look for free air.
   b. The sudden outpouring of gastroduodenal contents into the abdominal cavity produces one of the most dramatic clinical pictures encountered in surgery.
   c. The pain is sudden, reaches maximum intensity immediately and *remains* constant and unremitting.
   d. The patient has an anxious, pale appearance; the skin is wet with sweat, and the abdomen is held rigid. The patient does not move in bed at all.
   e. The rigidity is absolutely unyielding, resulting in the term "board-like."
   f. Peristaltic sounds are usually absent, and tenderness is most marked in the upper abdomen.
   g. The most reliable diagnostic procedure is x-ray demonstration of free intraperitoneal air. This can be demonstrated in approximately 85% of the patients, provided that upright and lateral decubitus films are made.

4. *Acute pancreatitis* is predominantly a disease of the obese and heavy drinker.
   a. It is characterized by a sudden onset of severe pain, usually following a large meal.
   b. The pain is quite severe, constant in character and radiates through to the back and always requires a narcotic for relief.
   c. The patient is obviously acutely ill; the abdomen may be soft, but tenderness and rebound tenderness are always present.
   d. Proper management of acute pancreatitis is not operative.
   e. The blood serum amylase is almost always elevated at some time during an episode of acute pancreatitis, especially in the early hours of the disease.
      1) The rise is frequently transitory and an

abnormal result may not be obtained; nevertheless the diagnosis cannot often be established clinically with certainty unless the serum or urine amylase value is known to be abnormal.

2) Many cases of pancreatitis either simulate or are associated with cholecystic disease and must be differentiated by means of laboratory tests.

5. The extra-abdominal causes of upper abdominal pain, such as *pneumonia, coronary occlusion* and *spontaneous pneumothorax,* are important considerations and should be kept in mind at all times.

IV. TRAUMATIC WOUNDS OF THE ABDOMEN

A. *Nonpenetrating* or blunt wounds of the abdomen may rupture a hollow viscus and cause peritonitis or may rupture a solid viscus and cause internal hemorrhage.

1. Many abdominal contusions occur without serious visceral damage, but the possibility of such injury must be kept in mind constantly and the patient examined at intervals of *1 or 2 hours* until a decision can be made regarding operation.

2. It is important to remember that a very trivial injury may *rupture* the bowel or spleen. The *consequences of* misdiagnosis are entirely out of proportion to the initial injury, and serious injuries may occur without a visible mark or contusion on the abdominal wall.

3. The diagnosis of blunt injury usually is not possible immediately after the accident because any severe blow on the abdomen causes sufficient disturbance to the nervous system to produce an early period of collapse.

4. Immediate laparotomy is, therefore, never advisable, because recovery from shock is frequently followed by spontaneous recovery from the trauma.

5. Difficulties in diagnosis arise because clinical evidence of injury may not appear until several hours later.

6. For this reason, it is mandatory that the *same physician* examine the patient at frequent intervals.
7. If intra-abdominal injury is suspected, transfusions should be given according to the patient's needs.
8. An intranasal gastric suction tube is inserted, a catheter is placed in the bladder and, as soon as the patient's condition permits, plain x-ray films of the abdomen in both supine and upright positions are made and examined for pneumoperitoneum or for a characteristic intestinal gas pattern. The absence of free intraperitoneal air *does not* rule out rupture of a hollow viscus.
9. In the absence of visceral injury, complete recovery should occur after a few hours.
10. A condition which simulates a serious intra-abdominal lesion but for which operation is not indicated is *adynamic ileus.*
11. It must be emphasized again that correct diagnosis depends to a great extent on the frequency and character of the clinical examinations.
12. Absolute indications for a laparotomy are:
    a. The presence of free intraperitoneal air.
    b. Abdominal paracentesis yields blood or intestinal content.
    c. The patient receives blood and recovers from initial shock, and then gradually the blood pressure slips lower, pallor increases and shock is again present. The clinical picture of progressive collapse after initial recovery is significant, since it cannot be ascribed to the shock of injury.
    d. In attempting to determine if there is internal blood loss, the red cell count, hemoglobin and hematocrit are *unreliable* in the *early* hours of massive hemorrhage.
13. Relative indications for laparotomy are:
    a. A gradual increase of abdominal distention with decreasing, and then absent, bowel sounds.
    b. Persistent abdominal tenderness even though present only with deep palpation.
14. Attempting to establish the exact diagnosis by

observation and re-examination *does not mean* that one should wait hours between examinations.

15. The *chance for successful treatment* is often passed if there is obvious peritonitis.

B. SPLEEN

1. Visceral injury occurs most often to the *spleen.*
2. Plain films of the abdomen are occasionally of considerable help in the diagnosis of splenic rupture.
3. Even small tears of the spleen continue to bleed, so that, once the diagnosis is made, splenectomy is indicated.
4. The typical picture of traumatic rupture of the spleen consists of:
   a. Abdominal pain.
   b. Tenderness.
   c. Evidence of internal hemorrhage.
5. Such a picture is considerably modified by the intensity and location of the hemorrhage, i.e., whether it is into the free peritoneal cavity or into a retroperitoneal space or into the spleen itself.
6. Delays and errors in diagnosis are usually caused by the failure to realize that these variations in pathology produce *marked variation* in the clinical signs. It is not uncommon to have a *slow leak* from the spleen, resulting in some *tenderness* in the left upper quadrant and a *persistent* low hematocrit despite transfusions.

C. Injury to the LIVER is about equally as common, but the bleeding may stop if the tear is small.

D. The BLADDER is the hollow viscus most frequently damaged.
   1. Injury is suspected in any patient with a *pelvic fracture* or in a patient in whom only a *few* drops of *bloody urine* are obtained by catheterization (see Chap. 16).

E. Abdominal paracentesis is performed by inserting a renal dialysis catheter below the umbilicus. A liter of physiologic saline is run in and then aspirated to determine if free blood exists in the peritoneal cavity.

1. A positive tap is helpful, but a *negative* tap does not rule out intra-abdominal injury and therefore other methods of diagnosis always must be used.

F. PENETRATING WOUNDS

1. These are usually produced by a knife or gunshot.
2. A problem in such wounds is to determine whether the *abdominal cavity* has been penetrated and, if so, what intra-abdominal structure has been injured.
3. There are *no insignificant* penetrating wounds of the abdomen.
   a. If the wound has *not* penetrated the peritoneum, local treatment in the Emergency Service without laparotomy is sufficient after recheck of vital signs and re-examinations by the same surgeon.
   b. A hemoglobin, hematocrit and urine examination are indicated. Repeat as needed.
4. An intranasal gastric tube, a catheter in the bladder and a rectal examination are indicated.
5. Upright and supine x-ray films are made to examine for pneumoperitoneum and for localization of the missile if the wound is from a bullet.
6. **Knife Wounds** seldom penetrate a viscus unless it is fixed; the organs tend to slide away from the advancing point of the knife.
   a. However, it is difficult to determine if an intra-abdominal structure has been damaged except by laparotomy.
   b. Interpret results by probing cautiously.
   c. *Presumptive* evidence of penetration of a viscus is:
      1) Abdominal tenderness and rebound tenderness.
      2) Increasing pulse rate, decreasing blood pressure.
      3) Rising hematocrit reading suggestive of internal hemorrhage.

d. *Obvious* evidence is:
   1) Pneumoperitoneum.
   2) Discharge of intestinal contents or bile from the wound.
   3) Blood from the stomach or bladder.

7. **Gunshot Wounds.**
   a. Unlike knife wounds, in which the viscera slip away from the path of the knife, a bullet rips through the abdomen and seriously damages all structures in its path.
   b. Massive peritoneal contamination or serious hemorrhage frequently results.
   c. The mortality rate from gunshot wounds of the abdomen is high and can be decreased only by *shortening the interval* between injury and operation.
   d. The time factor is crucial after gunshot wounds.
   e. Preoperative preparation as outlined for other penetrating wounds of the abdomen should be instituted immediately.
   f. Diagnostic effort is directed toward determining the exact course of the missile rather than weighing the evidence of penetration.
   g. Laparotomy is mandatory because of the serious nature of these wounds.
   h. A most important error is *failure* to examine the rectum.
   i. Injury to the rectum should be suspected in *all wounds* of the lower abdomen, buttock, sacrum and hip, especially if the wound of entry is on the posterior aspect of the thigh and the missile takes an *upward* course and has no point of exit.

V. MASSIVE GASTROINTESTINAL HEMORRHAGE

A. Patients with massive gastrointestinal hemorrhage present a most urgent problem and require immediate, accurate treatment.
   1. About two thirds of the patients with gastrointestinal

hemorrhage will have a peptic ulcer.
2. About 5% will bleed from gastric carcinoma or polyps.
3. Another 5% will have esophageal varices.
4. Severe bleeding from the *lower* gastrointestinal tract may be due to ulcerative colitis, bleeding diverticulosis, adenocarcinoma or large hemorrhoidal veins.
5. There is a large group of miscellaneous conditions which may cause severe bleeding. These include:
   a. Bleeding from the nose, mouth or respiratory passages.
   b. Hiatus hernia.
   c. Gastric lesions such as gastritis, foreign bodies, blood dyscrasias, etc.

B. A rapid history is taken, and inquiry should be made as to the use of steroids, salicylates, anticoagulants, as well as to hypertension.

C. The appearance of the blood may be helpful, since bright red blood results from profuse hemorrhage and little contact with gastric juice, whereas bleeding from the lower stomach or duodenum typically is "coffee ground" in appearance.

D. Evaluation of the patient includes:
   1. A search for signs and symptoms of cirrhosis (enlargement of the liver, spider nevi, palmar erythema and dilated superficial veins around the umbilicus).
   2. The identification of an esophageal varix as the source of bleeding is a palpable spleen, which will be present in two thirds of patients with hemorrhage from esophageal varices. A thin barium swallow will help.
   3. An abdominal mass, enlarged supraclavicular lymph nodes, a rectal shelf or an enlarged liver may indicate a gastric carcinoma.
   4. Examination of the rectum may show a tarry stool.
   5. Blood is taken for type and cross-match, and an intravenous catheter inserted.

6. I.V. fluid, oxygen and sedation are administered as indicated.
7. A nasogastric tube, which indicates the rate of bleeding and helps evacuate the stomach, is indicated.
8. *All* such patients should be *admitted* promptly, since a significant number will require emergency operation to control the hemorrhage.
    a. If the bleeding is due to esophageal varices, it usually will be necessary to pass a Patton or Sengstaken-Blakemore tube.
    b. After inflation of the balloons, traction must be maintained to hold the gastric baloon in place and-to maintain pressure against the bleeding point.
    c. If the bleeding arises from an *ulcer,* blood is replaced as indicated, and the patient is observed for evidence of persistence or continuation of the bleeding.
    d. If bleeding stops, the pressure and pulse rate tend to return to normal and evidence of shock will disappear.
    e. If bleeding persists, the return from the nasal tube will remain bright red, the pressure will remain low and symptoms of shock will persist.
    f. If bleeding persists and exceeds 500 ml. per 8-hour period, an emergency operation will be required.

CHAPTER 11

Management of Neurosurgical Problems

ERIC OLDBERG, M.D., *and*
OSCAR SUGAR, M.D.

I. HEAD INJURIES

A. Be sure the airway is clear.

B. Stop active bleeding by pressure unless a spurting vessel can be seen and clamped.

C. Investigate other parts of the body for life threatening injuries, (e.g., sucking wound of chest).

D. Do a brief but thorough *neurologic examination* and record as soon as possible.

   1. Evaluate the State of Consciousness.

   Changes in the state of consciousness are more important than all other examination findings in raising suspicion of intracranial hemorrhage.
   a. Is the patient awake?
   b. Does he answer questions and obey commands?
   c. If drowsy, can he be readily awakened?
   d. Is he oriented for time, place, and person?
   e. If unresponsive verbally, does he respond to painful stimuli such as pressure between mastoid and mandible or on supraorbital nerves or pinpricking of feet?
   f. If he moves, is the movement purposeful? (i.e., can respond to directions).
   g. Do all four extremities move?
   h. Is the movement restricted to flexion or extension of arms and legs (decerebrate response)?

2. **Examine the Eyes for Pupillary Size and Reaction to Light.**
   a. Unilateral enlargement of a pupil may indicate growing pressure in the head, especially when the patient is unresponsive.
   b. Fixed midsize or small pupils may mean a midbrain lesion.
   c. Pupillary inequality in the initial examination may be of no great concern if the patient is alert; if comatose, it may mean irretrievable damage.
   d. Fundoscopy in acute head injury is of little immediate importance and may be deferred, especially if the patient is restless or uncooperative.

3. **Eye Movement.**
   a. If the eyelids are not too swollen to prevent seeing the eye move, simple turning of eyes in response to command gives a baseline for recording.
   b. If the patient is unconscious, gently rotating the head to one side permits one to see if the eyeballs stay with the head (fixed) or move to the opposite side (doll's eyes phenomenon); movement indicates preservation of oculocephalic (proprioceptive headturning) reflex.

4. **Assessments of motor function** of jaws, face, palate and neck, readily done in conscious patients.

5. **Palpation of neck** posteriorly may permit recognition of dislocation or fracture and *must* precede any attempt to turn patient to examine the spine.

6. **Deep "Tendon" Reflexes.**
   a. May be elicited if time permits.
   b. Abdominal and cremasteric reflexes are not of immediate vital importance.
   c. Babinski or analogous signs *do* imply impairment of cerebrospinal pathways and should be tested.

7. **Bleeding from Ear and Nose.**
   a. Investigate to see if the source is from an adjacent laceration.

b. Admixture with cerebrospinal fluid, or leakage
of clear fluid by itself indicates *basal skull fracture regardless* of skull radiographs.

c. Prophylactic antibiotics and hospitalization for
observation are indicated.

d. If blood is present in ear canal or nose, do not
insert instruments, and do not try to dam up
with cotton or gauze. For cleanliness, gauze
can be taped against the external ear, still allowing otorrhea.

e. Obvious blood arising in the ear (e.g., bulging,
discolored eardrum) *also* indicates basal skull
fracture and hospitalization.

f. Nystagmus may be noted in the examination of
eye movements, and may mean cerebellar or
vestibular disturbance—or recent indulgence in
alcohol or other drugs.

g. Visual field testing may be useful in determining
possible optic nerve disorder.

h. Gait and coordination disturbances fall in this
same baseline category.

E. PENETRATING WOUNDS

1. The same procedures are used for penetrating wounds
(bullet, knife). If a knife or other foreign object pro-
trudes from the head, it should not be removed until
the neurosurgeon and craniotomy facilities are available.

2. Blood pressure, pulse, respiration recordings are
made at admission and at 30-60-minute intervals at
first, then at 1-4-hour intervals if the patient remains
comatose or the state of consciousness deteriorates.

3. Pupillary changes and responsiveness are also charted;
increase in pupil size, especially if unilateral, and decreasing level of alertness indicate *need for prompt*
neurosurgical attention.

4. Sedation obviously will interfere with these criteria
for alarm, and should be minimized. Aspirin (acetyl
salicylic acid) is useful for analgesia and may help

restlessness; if there is pain from an additional serious injury, narcotics may be necessary, but the mildest possible should be used.

5. If a convulsion occurs, anticonvulsants may be administered. Valium (diazepam), 10-15 mg. I.V., has the advantage of minimizing sedation, but sodium amytal 100-500 mg., I.V., may be needed. (See Chap. 17.)

6. Lumbar puncture is of little benefit in emergency care of patients with head injury, and should not be done unless a neurosurgical consultant so directs.

7. X-ray films of the head are rarely imperative in patients with severe closed head injuries; repeated clinical observations are more important. With missile injuries and compound fractures, location of bone and foreign objects becomes important and films are then needed. Care must be taken to consider injuries to the spine before twisting or turning the neck; when there is doubt, it is best to take just antero-posterior and across-the-table lateral views without turning the head. Finer details can wait for improvement in general state of the patient. When the patient is alert, and no serious neurologic problem exists, skull radiographs may be taken as part of the basis for making a decision as to release of the patient from the emergency room. The presence of a fracture is usually an indication of the severity of the head trauma and ordinarily indicates hospitalization for observation.

8. If echo-encephalography is available, its determination of the location of the midline echo may be a valuable indicator of the presence of a space-occupying mass inside the head, and hence alert neurosurgical consultation.

F. SCALP LACERATIONS

1. A generous area should be shaved (at least 3-4 cm.) around a laceration and copious amounts of saline or water used to wash out blood and dirt.

2. If there is active scalp bleeding, figure of eight or vertical mattress sutures are better than trying to apply hemostats to vessels smaller than superficial temporal, frontal or occipital arteries.
3. Before closure, the wound can be gently probed with sterile forceps or a sterile gloved finger to see if there is a fracture.
4. If a fracture is obvious, or if brain is extruding from the wound, repair should be done in the operating room as a formal procedure, *not* in the Emergency Room. If there is bleeding in such a compounded fracture, through and through sutures can stop it and these can be removed when the O.R. is ready.

II. SPINE INJURIES

A. Any patient who has fallen or who has been involved in an accident may have an injury to the spine and its contents. Consequently, a high index of suspicion is warranted for any unconscious patient brought into the Emergency Room, and movements should be gentle and guarded.

B. EXAMINATION

1. In the examination of the unconscious patient, the spine should be palpated from head to sacrum for obvious protrusions, malalignments, and areas from which palpation may evoke reflex pain withdrawal responses.
2. If the patient is to be turned, the head and body should be turned *en bloc* to avoid twisting the neck and spine until absence of injury is assured.
3. Determination of the presence of knee and ankle stretch reflexes and withdrawal responses to pin or other painful stimuli will aid even in the unconscious patient, for absence of such reflexes and responses may indicate "spinal shock," a condition in which synaptic conduction is depressed following gross insult to the spinal cord.
4. If the patient is conscious, neurologic examination

can rapidly detect spinal cord damage.
   a. Voluntary movement of the various parts of the
      extremities is requested.
   b. Reflexes are elicited (including plantar, abdom-
      inal, and cremasteric responses in males, biceps,
      triceps, knee, and ankle stretch reflexes. Re-
      sponses to pinprick also are elicited).
5. The level of spinal cord injury can be determined by
   the neurologic findings with reasonable accuracy in
   most cases (Tables 1 and 2).
   a. Most of the thoracic levels cannot be determined
      by muscular movements, except that forceful
      ventral flexion of the neck normally produces
      contraction of the recti abdomini muscles (T8-
      T12). If the umbilicus moves upward (Beevor's
      sign), the upper recti (T8-10) are active and the
      lower ones (T11-12) are not.

TABLE 1.–MOTOR LEVELS

Action	Muscles	Spinal Cord Levels
Shrugging shoulders	Trapezius	Accessory nerve, C2, C3
Flexion of forearm at elbow	Biceps	C5, 6
Extension of arm at elbow	Triceps	C6, 7
Ab- and adduction of fingers	Interossei and lumbricals	C8, T1
Flexion of thigh on abdomen	Iliopsoas	L1, 2, 3
Extension of lower leg at knee	Quadriceps	L2, 3, 4
Dorsiflexion of foot and great toe	Anterior tibial and peroneal muscles	L4, 5
Plantar flexion of foot	Gastrocnemius	L5, S1

TABLE 2.—SENSORY LEVELS

Area of Body	Spinal Cord Levels	Vertebral Body Levels
Neck to clavicle	C 2-4	C 2-4
Outer deltoid	C 5	C 5
Thumb	C 6	C 6
Index finger	C 7	C 7
Little finger	C 8	T 1
Nipple	T 3	T 2
Umbilicus	T 10	T 8
Inguinal area (groin)	L 1	T 10
Thigh above knee	L 3	T 11
Lateral calf	L 4	T 11-12
Foot dorsum	L 5	T 12
Lateral foot and small toe	S 1	L 1
Buttock	S 3-5	L 1-2

      b. In the cervical area, the vertebral bodies corres-
pond to the spinal cord segments; in the thoracic
region, the bodies are 1-2 segments higher than
the cord levels; the lumbar and sacral areas of the
cord are compressed at a level corresponding from
T 10 to the interspace between L 1 and L 2, where
the cord normally ends. Sensation for pin should
be checked on *both* sides of the body and also on
the back as well as front for discrepancies and
better localization.

    6. The most common serious injuries to the spine com-
patible with life are those at C 5-6, and those at
T 12-L 1.

      a. Lesions at or above C 4 usually involve phrenic
centers and apnea. Those at C 5-6 cause sensory
loss below the clavicles, and on the tricipital and
ulnar areas of the arm and hand.

    b.   Lesions at L 1 involve the conus medullaris, producing saddle anesthesia and sphincter loss.

    c.   Once the presumed locus of neurologic lesion is determined, radiographs of the spine corresponding to this area should be done. Movement of the patient with suspected spine lesion should be minimized, and hence complete x-ray examination may not be warranted.

    d.   Anteroposterior films can virtually always be done with the patient on the same table or cart on which he has been placed on entry into the Emergency Room: if other systemic injury does not forbid it, the patient should be taken to the x-ray department for these studies for the resulting films are superior to those done with most portable machines. A film-containing cassette can be placed under the patient and the tube moved over the patient rather than moving the patient onto the regular x-ray table.

    e.   Lateral films are best taken "across the table"; i.e., by holding a film alongside the neck (or body) and having the tube facing it across the patient's body, instead of turning the patient.

    f.   The area at C6-T1, especially in large males, may be difficult to visualize unless the arms are pulled down during the taking of the film, and oblique views, again without moving the patient, may be needed.

C.   TREATMENT

   1. If the films show fracture and or dislocation in the cervical spine, skull caliper traction should be immediately instituted wherever the patient is (X-ray Department, Emergency Room or Operating Room).

   2. Crutchfield or Vincke tongs are put in place in the parietal areas in line with the mastoid processes, and weights varying from 5-35 lbs. are put in place to help realign the bones (or to hold them in alignment).

3. Temporary halter traction may be used to help prevent further malalignment, and manual pulling on the halter may keep the neck in alignment while moving the patient in the hospital before tongs are available. If tongs are not immediately available, the head should be immobilized between sandbags.

4. If the patient is para- or quadriplegic, or if there is a lesion of the conus medullaris or cauda equina (implying bladder disability), the patient should be catheterized and the indwelling catheter (e.g., Foley) left in place attached by sterile tubing to a closed container.

5. After traction is instituted (or no need for it ascertained), the patient can be turned from side to side (by several persons, so that the neck and body will not be twisted) or from front to back on a turning frame. Frequent turning is by far the most effective way of preventing decubiti (bed sores).

6. If x-ray films show fractures of the neural arches, a decision will be needed concerning operation. Immediate neurosurgical consultation is required. Consultation is also required when there is a transverse lesion of the spinal cord or cauda equina *without* obvious bone lesion.

7. Lumbar puncture may be needed to determine the presence or absence of a spinal fluid block.

8. Emergency operation may be considered (diskectomy via anterior approach in the neck or laminectomy at any level of the spine).

9. When the films show obvious fracture-dislocation with neurologic deficit, spinal fluid block usually indicates necessity for operation, providing the general condition of the patient permits. Impairment of respiration takes precedence, as does evidence of bleeding in the abdomen or in the head.

10. Missile wounds and stab wounds of the spine with or without neurologic lesion ordinarily indicate formal operative intervention; protruding weapons should not be removed in the Emergency Room, nor should a bullet wound be probed. A pressure dressing may

be applied to minimize bleeding and the patient transported to the operating room with x-ray films taken in the Emergency Room, X-ray Department, or Operating Room as time and conditions indicate.

CHAPTER 12

Peripheral Vascular Emergencies

SIDNEY LEVITSKY, M.D., *and*
FREDERICK J. MERCHANT, M.D.

INTRODUCTION

The Emergency Service physician must realize that delay in the diagnosis and treatment of the patient with a peripheral vascular emergency may result in the loss of a limb.

Often, in a busy Emergency Service, the patient with limb pain is not immediately seen in favor of the patient with an obvious penetrating wound.

For this reason, *every* patient should be examined by a triage physician within minutes after arrival.

Although a nontraumatic peripheral vascular emergency appears obvious, there is often associated systemic disease. Therefore, the physician immediately must obtain a detailed history and perform a complete physical examination.

I. ACUTE ARTERIAL ISCHEMIA

A. EARLY SYMPTOMS AND SIGNS

1. Sudden onset of severe extremity pain.
2. Paresthesias followed by the gradual loss of sensation.
3. Gradual loss of motor function.
4. Coolness of the skin at a level compatible with the location of the anatomic obstruction.
   a. Aortic-iliac bifurcation—proximal to the knee.
   b. Common femoral—distal to the knee.
   c. Popliteal—distal third of leg.

5. Paleness of the extremity with diminished capillary filling of the toes.
6. Absence of pulses distal to the anatomic block.

B. LATE SYMPTOMS AND SIGNS

1. Violaceous hue of extremity.
2. Increase in size of extremity with firm consistency of muscles on palpation.
3. Dry or wet gangrene.
4. Gas gangrene.
5. Absence of pain or sensation in distal extremity.
6. Systemic bacteremia that may lead to septic shock.

II. TRAUMA

A. *Laceration, perforation* or *contusion* of the vessel wall may result in acute cessation of distal arterial flow.

B. If the artery is *completely severed,* the vessel retracts into the surrounding tissues. Usually, constriction of the open vessel edges by contraction of the circular coats of muscle in the media prevents extensive blood loss.

C. A *partially transected* major artery tends to gape widely and may result in severe hemorrhage.

D. *Arterial perforations* from knives, ice picks or low velocity missiles may not be apparent immediately if the surrounding tissues are filled with blood. However, if these injuries are untreated, arteriovenous fistulae or pulsating hematomas (false aneurysms) may result.

E. *Arterial contusions* commonly are caused by:
1. Crushing blunt trauma.
2. Fractures.
3. High velocity missiles passing in close proximity to the vessel.
   a. There is damage to the vessel wall with a hematoma developing between the intima and media.
   b. As the clot enlarges, the lumen of the vessel gradually becomes occluded (Fig. 12-1).

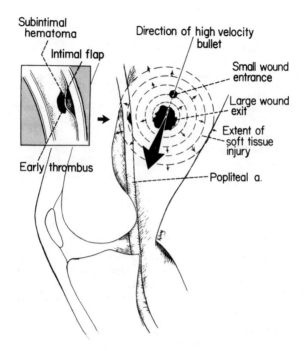

Fig. 12-1.—Arterial injury in lower thigh due to high velocity missile.

F. Arterial injuries are also associated with supracondylar fractures of the humerus and femur (Fig. 12-2).

G. In rapid decelerating automobile and airplane accidents, the *origin* of the *left subclavian artery* may be subjected to a shearing force; an absent left radial pulse may be the first indication of injury to the descending thoracic aorta.

H. **Treatment**
　　1. Initial.
　　　　a. Local control of hemorrhage.

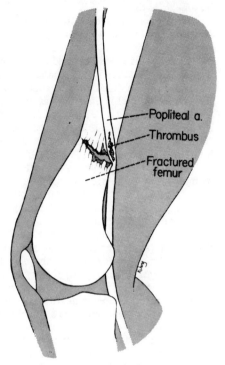

Fig. 12-2.—Popliteal artery injury associated with a supracondylar fracture of the femur.

     b. Resuscitation of the patient.
  2. The patient should not be anesthetized unless there is a severe intra-abdominal or intrathoracic hemorrhage.
  3. Intravascular volume must be restored and hypoxemia and acidosis corrected.
  4. *Arterial bleeding* from a limb wound usually can be controlled by bulky compression dressings reinforced

by an elastic bandage.

5. Under *no* circumstances should one attempt to control bleeding by blindly clamping in the depths of the wound.
   a. Tourniquets should be used only if *absolutely necessary* as they occlude collateral circulation and promote distal intravascular thrombosis.
   b. If a tourniquet is the only way to stop the bleeding, it *must* be loosened *every 20 minutes.*

6. *Fractures* should be *stabilized* by splinting before transportation of the patient to avoid additional injury to adjacent vessels.

7. Preliminary arteriography to show the exact point of injury may be helpful, but is not absolutely necessary.

8. If there is any question of arterial integrity, the patient should undergo arterial exploration.

9. Exploration is also *mandatory* if a high velocity missile penetrates an area adjacent to a major vessel.

10. A detailed discussion of the techniques of arterial repair is beyond the scope of this manual. However, all procedures should be performed in a major operating room where adequate anesthesia, light, instruments and assistance are available. Basic principles include:
    a. Proximal and distal vessel control.
    b. Regional heparinization.
    c. Adequate debridement of vessel edges and adjacent tissue.

III. EMBOLI

A. Most arterial emboli arise from intracardiac thrombus formations. *Atrial fibrillation, mitral stenosis* or a recent *myocardial infarction* are frequently associated with thrombi.

B. Rarely, a left atrial *myxoma* may present as an acute arterial embolus; an argument for routine histologic study of all extracted clots.

C. The *embolus* commonly lodges at major vessel bifurcations (Fig. 12-3).

D. The pulse above a distal extremity obstruction is usually stronger than a pulse in the normal contralateral limb.

E. *Arteriography* may be useful in anatomic localization and in the elderly may reveal associated obstruction secondary to *arteriosclerosis obliterans.*

Fig. 12-3.—Aorto-iliac embolus originating in a left ventricular myocardial infarction.

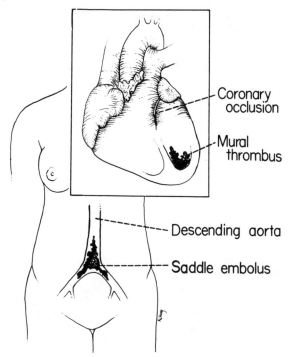

F. Surgical intervention should *not* be delayed if arteri-
    ography is not available immediately.

G. As soon as the *diagnosis* is made, the patient should be
    given heparin, (50-75 mg. I.V. for an adult) to prevent
    distal intravascular thrombosis.

H. **Treatment** is directed toward expeditious extraction of
    the clot.
    1. In most patients, the procedure can be performed
        under local anesthesia.
    2. The development of the balloon tip catheter has
        greatly facilitated the ease with which emboli can
        be removed.
    3. Retrograde transfemoral extraction of an aortic-iliac
        saddle embolus can be performed under local anes-
        thesia.

IV. ARTERIOSCLEROSIS OBLITERANS

A. Occlusion in this arterial disease of aging is a gradual,
    progressive process.

B. It is usually accompanied by the development of collat-
    eral circulation.

C. Occasionally, the narrow vessel lumen will thrombose
    suddenly causing acute ischemia.

D. The patient often presents with a history and signs and
    symptoms of:
    1. Leg claudication.
    2. Trophic skin changes.
    3. Ulceration.
    4. Areas of gangrene.

E. **Management**
    1. As soon as the *diagnosis* is made, the patient should
        be given heparin (50-75 mg. I.V. for an adult) and
        admitted to the hospital. Sympathetic block and
        drugs promoting vasodilatation have little or no ef-
        fect on diseased arteriosclerotic vessels.
    2. Arrangements should be made for immediate arteri-
        ography.

3. The patient should be *evaluated frequently* (2-3-hour intervals).

4. If there is *proximal progression* of skin coolness, evidence of a *decrease in motor activity* or *sensation, immediate* surgical intervention is necessary.

5. Many of these elderly patients have diseases involving multiple systems and represent a substantial risk for what is usually a long surgical procedure. Therefore, it is best to operate on these patients *electively* following thorough preoperative evaluation.

F. Operative procedures include endarterectomy or the insertion of bypass grafts of autogenous tissue or synthetic material.

V. ACUTE VENOUS PROBLEMS

A. TRAUMA

1. Major vein injury usually is associated with arterial trauma. Occasionally, however, a penetrating wound may involve only a large vein.

2. As in arterial trauma, active bleeding is controlled by compression dressings; blind clamping in the depths of the wound is to be *avoided*.

3. Recent experience with Vietnam battle casualties following traumatic injury to major extremity veins has indicated that direct repair of the vein, if possible, is preferable to ligation.

4. Since direct repair of injured veins has been introduced, the incidence of posttraumatic extremity edema and phlebitis has markedly decreased.

B. RUPTURED VARICOSITIES

1. Hemorrhage of a thin, dilated superficial vein in patients with varicose veins of the lower extremity may occur spontaneously or following traumatic injury.

2. The area where the greater saphenous vein crosses the medial malleolus is most commonly involved (Fig. 12-4).

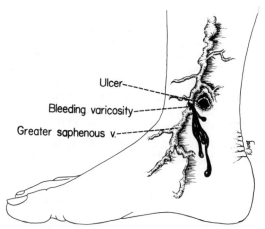

Fig. 12-4.—Fragile varicosity associated with a stasis ulcer.

3. Blood loss is usually minimal but may be extensive
    enough to require transfusion. Bleeding is easily
    controlled by direct application of a compression
    dressing followed by an elastic bandage from the
    toes to the tibial tubercle.
4. Subcutaneous and intradermal rupture of a varix
    results in an ecchymotic patch or hematoma, which
    if untreated, can lead to a stasis ulcer.

C. THROMBOPHLEBITIS

1. *Acute superficial thrombophlebitis* occurs:
    a. Spontaneously in patients with varicose veins.
    b. In women during and following pregnancy.
    c. Following chemical and mechanical trauma.
    d. In patients with carcinoma or blood dyscrasias.
    e. The lesions present as painful, erythematous
        cords following the course of superficial veins.
        The inflammatory reaction usually subsides in
        7-18 days.

f. **Treatment** includes:
1) Bedrest with elevation of the extremity.
2) Warm, moist packs and analgesics.
3) If there is involvement of the *deep* venous system, anticoagulation therapy is indicated (heparin, 50 mg. I.V., every 4 hours).
4) Antibiotic administration is indicated only if *suppurative* phlebitis is present.

2. **Deep Thrombophlebitis.**
a. The *urgent nature* of this condition stems from the often fatal complication of pulmonary embolism.
b. Thrombophlebitis most commonly involves the deep veins of the calves, the iliofemoral system, the pelvic veins and the axillary vein.
c. Venous stasis is the underlying cause of deep thrombophlebitis.
d. *Other factors* include:
1) Trauma.
2) Postoperative and postpartum states.
3) Blood dyscrasias.
4) Carcinoma, particularly of the pancreas and prostate.
5) Heart failure.
e. Recently, it has been suggested that smoking and the administration of oral contraceptives are related to hypercoagulability, thus setting the stage for the phlebitic process.
f. **Signs and Symptoms.**
1) There is usually a *rapid onset* of pain and swelling of the limb.
2) Diffuse muscular tenderness on manual compression.
3) Forcible dorsiflexion of the foot causes pain in the calf (Homans' sign) in the early stages of the disease.
4) In subclinical cases, *calf tenderness* on palpation and a *firmness* of the calf muscles may be the only signs.

5) Iliofemoral thrombophlebitis causes swelling of the thigh and tenderness along the common femoral vein beneath the inguinal ligament.
6) The calf and thigh circumferences of the involved extremity may exceed a normal contralateral extremity by 2 cm.

3. Phlegmasia Cerulea Dolens.

a. This is a severe form of iliofemoral thrombophlebitis and is secondary to thrombosis of the major tributaries of the femoral vein.
b. It is associated with:
   1) Marked swelling.
   2) Cyanosis.
   3) Petechiae.
   4) Ecchymotic patches.
c. The arterial blood supply may become secondarily obstructed from edema and *gangrene* may occur.
d. In rare cases, in the elderly with contracted blood volumes, the trapping of large volumes of blood in the limb may result in *hypovolemic shock*.
e. **Immediate Therapy.**
   1) Elevation of the foot of the bed on 6-inch wooden blocks with avoidance of flexion at the trunk and inguinal region.
   2) Anticoagulation with heparin (50 mg. I.V. every 4 hours).
   3) Analgesics.
   4) Hydration.
   5) Low molecular weight Dextran I.V. (500-1000 ml./24 hours) may relieve pain and decrease venous stasis in some patients.
f. Regional sympathetic block and fasciotomy have *not* been helpful.
g. Thrombectomy has been reported to hasten symptomatic relief; whether it will decrease the incidence of chronic venous sufficiency has not been settled.

CHAPTER 13

Treatment of Burns

JOHN A. BOSWICK, JR., M.D.

I. GENERAL PRINCIPLES

A. One of the most difficult experiences that an Emergency Room physician may experience is the management of the severely burned patient. This is especially true if the patient is a child accompanied by frightened and apprehensive parents.

B. It is important that every physician should be able to decide which patient requires hospitalization, what therapy can safely be instituted in the Emergency Service and which patient requires certain initial procedures before being sent to his room or ward in the hospital.

C. Rigid asepsis (cap, mask, gown, instruments, gloves, etc.) must be the rule in evaluating and treating the patient with a thermal injury. Until some type of therapy is instituted, the wounds are open and subject to contamination.

D. The initial step in evaluating and managing a burn patient is a detailed, thorough history and physical examination. While detailed and thorough, it should be done rapidly, requiring no more than 15 or 20 minutes.

E. The history should include the place and cause of injury in detail and the type and time of any care rendered before reaching the hospital. Any pre-existing disease that might influence the course and care of the patient, i.e., cardiac, renal, metabolic and other disorders, must be ascertained.

F. A complete and thorough medical examination is basic, including vital signs and an accurate as possible estimation as to the extent and depth of injury.

G. These are best made after initial wound care has been performed. A rough estimation as to the extent and depth of burn is helpful at this point to determine whether the patient requires hospitalization and intravenous fluid therapy. A standard or uniform technique for measuring or estimating the extent and depth of the burn should be employed at every hospital (Fig. 13-1).

Fig. 13-1.–How to estimate percentage of burn.

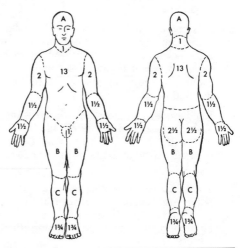

Relative percentage of areas affected by growth	AGE IN YEARS					
	0	1	5	10	15	adult
Partial Thickness – Blue A—½ of head	9½	8½	6½	5½	4½	3½
Full Thickness – Red B—½ of one thigh	2¾	3¼	4	4¼	4½	4¾
C—½ of one leg	2½	2½	2¾	3	3¼	3½
Total per cent burned	———— Partial ———— Full ————					

II. MINOR BURNS—INITIAL CARE

A. Partial thickness or questionable depth burns involving the extremities and trunk other than the hand or face can often be treated safely on an outpatient basis.

B. If such a patient is seen early after injury and the wound is located where cold packs can be applied or the part can be immersed in ice water, this is excellent technique for relieving pain and possibly preventing edema formation. We have found it most useful in the extremity.

C. It is best to use this technique after the wound has been cleansed with soap and water and the blisters broken and loose tissue excised.

D. If pain or edema does not appear to be a problem in a minor wound, dressings are indicated to protect the wound from further trauma or contamination.

E. One of the most satisfactory dressings in this situation is saline-moistened fine-mesh gauze next to the wound followed by three or four layers of saline-moistened coarse mesh gauze. This is followed by several layers of cut and fluffed coarse gauze held in place by Cohesive.

F. Too much compression must be avoided. The application of an elastic bandage over such a dressing is *not* recommended.

III. SEVERITY OF INJURY

A. While there is no completely accurate way of classifying every patient as to minor, moderate or severe burns, there are certain helpful guides.

B. Most burns over 20-25% of the body surface that have some portion of full thickness elements should be considered severe.
   1. Most patients with burns of the hand, face, feet or perineum should be considered to be severely burned because of the anatomic location.
   2. Burns of 10 or 15% in the patient over 60 or 65 years of age and in an infant under a year and a half

should be classified as severe burns. Patients in the extremes of age do not tolerate a thermal injury as well as a healthy young adult.

3. Electrical and chemical burns should also be considered severe injuries. The exact extent and depth of these injuries is difficult to estimate for many days after the injury.

4. Patients with renal, cardiac, or metabolic diseases, such as diabetes, can show a complicated response to injury and make therapy more difficult. Their burns should also be considered severe, in order that intensive care may be given.

IV. EXTENT OF BURN

A. The extent of every thermal injury should be recorded on an appropriate diagram or chart and made a part of the permanent record of the patient (see Fig. 13-1).

B. We find it useful to re-evaluate the extent of a burn injury 3 *weeks* after admission to the hospital or injury and *again on discharge* from the hospital. Appraisals of this type allow us to evaluate our ability to estimate whether a burn is partial or full thickness in depth.

V. DEPTH OF INJURY

A. Even an experienced surgeon will have difficulty in diagnosing the depth of a burn injury, as many burns cannot accurately be diagnosed for several days after the injury.

B. Two of the most helpful guides in this regard are the history of injury and the appearance of the wound.

C. The majority of patients sustaining thermal injury due to scalding, that is, burning with hot liquids, will have only partial thickness wounds.

D. Thermal injuries caused by flame, electricity, or contact with hot metal, conversely, will have, in most cases, partial full thickness wounds.

VI. URGENT MEASURES

A. *Tracheostomy.*—Certain patients with burns will require tracheostomy to maintain a patent airway. The indications for tracheostomy in the burn patient are similar to those in any traumatized patient.
1. Closure of the upper airway in the burn patient, that is, the nasal pharynx, is usually due to burn wound edema.
2. Some patients with burns will be so severely traumatized that they cannot handle their secretions without a tracheostomy.
3. Patients with deep burns about the face and neck and where there is indication of respiratory tract damage from smoke inhalation, often require tracheostomy.

B. *Fluid Resuscitation.*—Every severely burned patient should have initial fluid administration planned by using an acceptable burn formula. There are many good formulas for this purpose, but one we find very satisfactory is that adopted by Doctor Evans. General fluid resuscitation should be individualized, especially after the first 24-hour period.

VII. FLUID REQUIREMENTS (EVANS)

First 24 Hours.

Plasma: 1 ml./kg. body weight/% burn (up to 50%).

Saline: 1 ml./kg. body weight/% burn (up to 50%).

Glucose, 5%: 2000 ml. Give one half of total during first 8 hours after burn.

After First 24 Hours.

Guides:
1. Urine output: Optimum; 25-50 ml. per hour. Measure the specific gravity.
2. Clinical signs: Temperature, pulse rate, blood pressure, etc.

A. It must be stressed that overhydration is tolerated poorly by infants, young children and the aged. Fluids also must be administered cautiously in patients with borderline cardiac, pulmonary and renal reserves. All burned patients must be re-evaluated frequently to ensure accurate fluid intake.

B. A burn of more than 50% is considered as 50% for purposes of fluid therapy, since the amount of fluid lost does not increase greatly with the greater injury.

C. An alternate method of fluid replacement is the use of Lactated Ringers Solution, 4 ml./kg. of body weight per per cent burn. Plasma will be needed in the early post-burn period. The use of whole blood will depend upon hematocrit and hemoglobin levels after the patient is stabilized.

D. The Brooke formula is equally satisfactory.

VIII. WOUND CARE

A. While the management of the burn wound itself is not as urgent as airway patency, fluid resuscitation or the administration of antibiotics, it should be considered a part of the initial management of the burn patient. After urgent measures have been instituted and the patient has been given adequate analgesics in order that wound care can be given, the following steps should be performed.
    1. The wound should be washed thoroughly and gently with soap and water; there should be no time limit on this. All dirt and debris should be removed.
    2. If the wound involves hair-bearing areas, they should be gently shaved.
    3. All blisters should be broken, evacuated, and trimmed.
    4. All loose tissue should be gently but completely excised, using tissue forceps and scissors.

B. There is a difference of opinion concerning whether an antibacterial solution should be applied to the burn

wound or whether it should be left exposed to the air
or covered with a voluminous dressing.

C. We believe that some antibacterial agent is indicated for
deep partial and full thickness burn wounds. Sulfamylon
cream is most effective when properly used. Others have
reported good experience using a dilute (0.5) silver nitrate solution.

D. Some believe that washing the wound, keeping it free
from exudate and crust formation and applying a topical
solution of antibiotics is the only therapy required.

E. In burns of 15-20% or greater, the use of Penicillin G. is
effective in preventing burn wound cellulitis. The use
of other systemic antibiotics must be individualized.

F. If transportation of a patient involves a long distance or
requires several hours, a voluminous dressing is quite
helpful in reducing pain and preventing contamination
of the wound.

IX. ADDITIONAL FACTORS

A. If the patient is not at his regular weight, he should be
weighed shortly after admission to the hospital. This is
helpful in evaluating and planning therapy initially, and
also in evaluating nutritional requirement in the early,
intermediate and post-burn periods.

B. Most patients with extensive burns have paralytic ileus
often accompanied by gastric dilatation. Therefore,
they should not be fed until there are adequate bowel
sounds and other indications that they can tolerate oral
feedings.

C. Adequate records must be initiated immediately in addition to the one that estimates the extent and depth of
burn.
   1. Urinary output should be recorded, along with frequent hematocrits and other vital signs.
   2. An accurate intake record should also be maintained
   recording the type and quantity of fluid administered.

D. If there are definite indications of gastric dilatation by abdominal distention or vomiting, a nasal gastric tube should be inserted immediately.

E. Multiple vitamins should be given to most severely burned patients, including at least 1-1½ Gm. of vitamin C daily.

F. Both analgesics and barbiturates should be avoided wherever possible.

G. Burn wound cultures always are indicated.

H. Families of severely burned patients should be notified of their condition; the patient is placed on the critical list.

I. In extensively burned patients, frequent laboratory data, including hematocrit, hemoglobin, BUN and electrolytes, are needed.

J. It should be remembered that there are no strict rules for managing the severely burned patient. All therapy is based on the initial evaluation and close scrutiny of the patient on a day-to-day basis. The best surgeon for managing the severely burned patient is one who is humble enough to seek consultation when there is the slightest indication it is needed.

CHAPTER 14

Common Medical Emergencies

ROBERT C. MUEHRCKE, M.D.

I. GENERAL CONSIDERATIONS

The patient with an acute medical emergency must have accurate clinical appraisal with rapid institution of effective treatment. Prompt and intelligent management of the patient may result not only in the saving of life, but also in the prevention of a prolonged disability and in the arrest of further deterioration of a specific body function. (See Chap. 1, "Cardiopulmonary Resuscitation.")

II. RAPID APPRAISAL OF THE PATIENT

A. **HISTORY** (from the patient, family, friends, police, firemen, ambulance drivers, bystanders).

1. **Present Illness.**
   a. Onset.
   b. Infection.
   c. Contacts.
   d. Foul play.
   e. Progressions.
   f. Treatment.
   g. Sequelae.

2. **Past Illnesses.**
   a. Previous episodes.
   b. Chronic illness.
   c. Medications.
   d. Allergy.

3. **Examination of Patient's Personal Effects.**
   a. Clothing.

    b. Identification cards.
    c. Medical cards for diabetes mellitus.
    d. Epilepsy.
    e. Anticoagulants.
    f. Adrenal corticosteroids.

B. PHYSICAL EXAMINATION (Remove all clothing, cut free if necessary.)

  1. General Appearance.
    a. Asphyxia.
    b. Cyanosis.
    c. Pallor.
    d. Hemorrhage.
    e. Pulse rate.
    f. Blood pressure.
    g. Temperature.
    h. Orientation.
    i. Skin.
    j. Jaundice.
    k. Movement of limbs.

  2. Head.
    a. Nuchal rigidity.
    b. Pupils and eye muscles.
    c. Ears or nose.
    d. Position of trachea.
    e. Neck-vein distention.

  3. Chest.
    a. Sucking wounds.
    b. Crush injury.
    c. Auscultation.
    d. Rib fracture.
    e. Fluid.
    f. Murmurs.
    g. Cardiac rate and rhythm.
    i. Heart size.

  4. Abdomen.
    a. Masses.

    b. Ecchymosis.
    c. Abdominal vein.
    d. Pulsating masses.
    e. Fluid.
    f. Tenderness.
    g. Organ enlargement.
    h. Bladder fullness.
    i. Pain.
    j. Muscle spasm.

5. **Back.**
    a. Ecchymosis.
    b. Swelling.
    c. Tenderness.
    d. Spine.
    e. Kidney tenderness.
    f. Flank fullness.

6. **Extremities.**
    a. Movement.
    b. Color.
    c. Edema.
    d. Deformity.
    e. Needle punctures.
    f. Tenderness of fracture.

7. **Neurologic.**
    a. Orientation.
    b. Muscle rigidity.
    c. Muscle activity.
    d. Reflexes.
    e. Sensations.
    f. Stimulation.

III. CLASSIFICATION OF COMMON MEDICAL EMERGENCIES

The following outlines the prompt appraisal and treatment of the patient with the more common medical emergencies. No attempt is made to outline therapeutic measures after immediate medical emergency care. Patients brought to the

Emergency Service as medical emergencies usually can be *classified* in one of the following groups:

A. COMA

1. Meningitic.
2. Diabetic.
3. Hypoglycemic.
4. Uremic.
5. Hepatic.
6. Drug or poison induced.
7. Head trauma.
8. Alcoholic.
9. Addisonian crisis.
10. Hypertensive encephalopathy, etc.

B. NEUROLOGIC AND MUSCULAR DISORDERS

1. Acute cerebral vascular accidents and space-occupying lesions.
2. Acute convulsive disorders.
3. Myasthenia gravis.

C. INTOXICATIONS

1. Poisons.
2. Gases.
3. Drugs.

D. CARDIOVASCULAR DISORDERS

1. Shock.
2. Cardiac arrest.
3. Acute dysrhythmias.
4. Acute myocardial infarction.
5. Acute pulmonary edema.

E. PULMONARY DISORDERS

1. Asphyxia.
2. Bronchial asthma.
3. Acute respiratory acidosis.

4. Acute pneumonia.
5. Pulmonary embolism.

F. GASTROINTESTINAL DISORDERS

1. Acute nonsurgical abdomen.
2. Acute gastroenteritis.

G. EXPOSURE AND THERMAL INJURY

1. Electric shock.
2. Heatstroke or sunstroke.
3. Heat exhaustion.
4. Cold injury (frostbite).
5. Decompression sickness.

H. DRUG REACTIONS

1. Anaphylactic (allergic) shock.
2. Urticaria (hives) and angioneurotic edema.
3. Exfoliative dermatitis and serum sickness.

IV. MANAGEMENT OF COMA

A. The *general therapeutic principles* concerning the patient in coma are as follows:
1. Maintain pulmonary ventilation.
2. Arrest bleeding and control shock.
3. Insert intravenous plastic tube (Intra-Cath) for administration of fluids or medication.
4. Control temperature by use of:
   a. Aspirin.
   b. Rectal suppositories.
   c. Tepid-water sponging.
   d. Cold-water mattress.
   e. Chlorpromazine.
   f. Alcohol sponging.
   g. Propeller fan.
5. Insert a Foley catheter.
6. Prevent corneal ulcers.

B. TREATMENT OF SPECIFIC TYPES OF COMA

1. Meningitic Coma.

a. Symptoms and signs are:
1) Previous contact.
2) Severe headache.
3) Fever.
4) Prior confusion.
5) Stiff neck.
6) Petechia.
7) Purpuric rash.

b. **Treatment.**
1) Isolation procedures are used. Treatment for *shock and adrenal insufficiency* should be started before proceeding with definitive care.
2) A lumbar puncture usually is done in the Emergency Service and the cerebral spinal fluid rushed to the laboratory for bacterial smear, culture, cell count, protein and glucose values.
3) An *intravenous* route is established for the subsequent administration of antibiotics.
4) Hospitalize immediately.
5) Other members of the family and Emergency Service personnel may require prophylactic sulfonamide therapy.

2. Diabetic Coma.

a. Symptoms and signs are:
1) Kussmaul breathing.
2) Acetone breath.
3) Dehydration.
4) Shock.
5) Glycosuria.
6) Acetonuria.

b. **Treatment.**
1) Blood is drawn for chemical analysis (glucose, blood urea nitrogen, carbon dioxide, sodium and potassium).

2) The *urine* is examined for specific gravity, glucose, protein, cells, casts and ketone bodies.

3) Intravenous fluids are started (5% glucose in 1/2 normal saline solution with added sodium bicarbonate 44 or 88 mEq.—avoid lactate solutions).

4) *Regular insulin* is given intravenously (50-100 units).

5) *Shock* should be managed with vasopressive agents.

6) The condition of so-called "syrup diabetes" should not be missed. The patient may have had previous episodes of convulsions and enter the Emergency Service confused.

   a) He may have massive glycosuria, acetonuria and a very elevated blood glucose level, usually more than 1000 mg./100 ml.

   b) The CO_2 combining power may be near normal or normal.

   c) *Treatment* consists of prompt and effective administration of hypotonic fluids in massive amounts.

   d) Large quantities of regular insulin are given intravenously and subcutaneously.

   e) It may be necessary to insert a gastric tube and administer large quantities of water.

3. Hypoglycemic Shock.

a. Symptoms and signs are:
   1) Headache.
   2) Nervousness.
   3) Weakness.
   4) Sweating.

b. **Treatment.**
   1) Blood is drawn for glucose determinations.
   2) Fifty ml. of 50% glucose solution is given intravenously. Glucagon, 1 mg., has been

found to be effective in emergency therapy.
3) *Shock* should be managed with vasopressive agents. After the patient is stable, *hospitalize.*
4) Patients *not in shock* with hyperinsulinism usually are discharged and referred to the family physician for follow-up care.

4. **Uremic Coma.**
   a. Symptoms and signs.
      1) Physical findings of pallor, hypertension, urinous odor, uremic frost or twitching and funduscopic findings of retinitis may be present.
      2) If the patient deteriorates acutely, the physician must suspect one of the following:
         a) Sodium depletion.
         b) Congestive heart failure.
         c) Drug-induced hypovolemia.
         d) Acute pyelonephritis.
         e) Sudden severe hypertension.
   b. **Treatment.**
      1) As the patient is being evaluated, an airway is maintained.
      2) Sodium phenobarbital is given I.V., slowly, for convulsions. Dilantin is also effective, I.V., then orally.
      3) Antihypertensive agents, such as parenteral Hyperstat, Serpasil, Arfonad, Aldomet, or hydralazine, are used to lower the blood pressure.
      4) I.V. dextrose with or without sodium chloride and sodium bicarbonate may be given to correct acidosis.

5. **Hepatic Coma.**
   a. Symptoms and signs are:
      1) Jaundice.
      2) Ascites.
      3) Spider nevi.
      4) Palmar erythema.

     5) Dark urine.

     6) Flapping tremor.

     7) Flaccid paralysis.

     8) Hepatic coma is usually precipitated by a sedative, hemorrhage, a narcotic, alcohol, high-protein feedings and excessive use of oral diuretics.

  b. **Treatment.**

     1) Oxygen and I.V. fluids are started in the Emergency Service. These should include multivitamins and broad-spectrum antibiotics. Adrenal corticosteroids may be advisable.

     2) One should evaluate the patient with hepatic coma for hypoglycemia, infection, hemorrhage and hypokalemia.

6. **Drug or Poison-Induced Coma** (see Chap. 20).

7. **Head Trauma** (see Chap. 11).

8. **Alcoholic Coma.**

  a. In severe alcoholic coma, death is likely to occur from respiratory arrest, hypostatic pneumonia or increasing intracranial pressure.

  b. If the patient is in "light" alcoholic coma, he can, in some instances, be returned to his home after Emergency Service care.

  c. If he has had convulsions or if delirium tremens is present, he should be admitted to the hospital, for this is the most dramatic and grave of all alcoholic complications with the exception of Wernicke's encephalopathy.

  d. I.V. fluids containing glucose, multivitamins, magnesium salts and small dosages of regular insulin should be started.

  e. The stomach should be aspirated. An adequate airway should be maintained. The patient should be kept warm.

  f. β-ethyl-methylzutramide (Meziomide) may be given for severe respiratory depression.

9. **Addisonian Crisis.**
   a. The immediate treatment of the patient with addisonian crisis may be lifesaving.
   b. Acute adrenal insufficiency is manifested by shock, dehydration, fever and hypoglycemia. Confirmation of the diagnosis cannot be made while the patient is in shock.
   c. Therapy is directed to the elimination of the predisposing cause—restore the plasma and extracellular fluid volume and correct the hypoglycemia.
   d. Blood is drawn for determinations of sodium, potassium, urea nitrogen, chloride and carbon dioxide.
   e. An Intra-Cath is inserted, and 100 mg. of Solu-Cortef is given immediately. This is followed by 5% glucose in normal saline solution with additional adrenal corticosteroid added.
   f. Quarter-hourly recordings are made of blood pressure, fluid intake, urine output, temperature and pulse. The patient is admitted to the Medical Service for further therapy and evaluation.

10. **Hypertensive Encephalopathy.**
    a. This is usually associated with malignant hypertension. The blood pressure is greatly elevated and papilledema is found.
    b. Parenteral hypotensive medication should be used, (reserpine, 2.5 mg., I.M. with hydralazine, 20 mg.). Trimethaphan camphorsulfonate (Arfonad), in 500 ml. of 5% dextrose and infused at a rate of 10 drops (0.5 mg.) per minute. The rate of infusion may be increased depending upon the patient's response.
    c. Intravenous Aldomet, 500 mg. in one liter of 5% glucose can be beneficial.

11. **Coma from Other Causes.**
    a. Febrile illness.
    b. Brain tumor.
    c. Encephalitis.

    d. Heatstroke.
    e. Chronic subdural hematoma.

V. MANAGEMENT OF NEUROLOGIC AND MUSCULAR DISORDERS

A. ACUTE CEREBRAL VASCULAR ACCIDENTS

1. There are five major forms of acute cerebral vascular afflictions producing an acute brain syndrome:
   a. Cerebral infarction.
   b. Cerebral hemorrhage.
   c. Cerebral embolism.
   d. Intermittent cerebral ischemic attacks (internal carotid artery syndrome and basilar-vertebral artery system syndrome).
   e. Primary subarachnoid hemorrhage (from ruptured aneurysm).
2. In addition, one must consider space-occupying lesions such as primary or metastatic brain tumors and brain abscess.
3. Supportive therapy should be instituted: maintain an airway and support circulation with adequate fluids and electrolytes.

B. ACUTE CONVULSIVE DISORDERS

See Chapter 17, "Management of Convulsive Disorders."

C. MYASTHENIA GRAVIS

1. This disorder is characterized by weakness and marked fatigability of the voluntary muscles. Recovery from weakness or fatigue occurs with rest and specific medications.
2. Patients may suddenly develop inability to swallow or a respiratory crisis.
3. Neostigmine methylsulfate, 0.5 mg., is given subcutaneously or intramuscularly if severe symptoms develop.

4. Should respiratory distress develop, oxygen, intra-tracheal suction, mechanical positive-pressure respirators (Bennett) and tracheostomy are useful. In all instances, the patient should be admitted to the Medical Ward.
5. Patients who survive a crisis may have a remission lasting for several years.
6. Other neurologic and muscular diseases involving the respiratory muscles include the Guillain-Barre syndrome and progressive muscular dystrophy.

VI. MANAGEMENT OF INTOXICATION

See Chapter 20, "Management of Poisoning."

VII. MANAGEMENT OF CARDIOVASCULAR DISORDERS

The medical emergencies of cardiovascular disorders are divided into five groups: shock, cardiac arrest, acute dysrhythmias, acute myocardial infarction and acute pulmonary edema.

A. **SHOCK** (see Chap. 1, "Cardiopulmonary Resuscitation").

B. **CARDIAC ARREST** (see Chaps. 1 and 2).

C. **ACUTE DYSRHYTHMIAS**
1. The electrocardiogram will be the most helpful diagnostic aid in differentiating and distinguishing the various dysrhythmias.
2. Many Emergency Services contain portable battery-operated cardioscopes that are useful in the continuing monitoring of a patient with an acute dysrhythmia.
3. Particular attention should be given to drug ingestion (digitalis), potassium deficiency due to oral diuretic agents, a history of an acute myocardial

infarction, pulmonary embolism, hyperthyroidism and pulmonary infections.

4. The selection of treatment is based on the urgency of the clinical situation.

5. **Regular Dysrhythmias.**
   a. If the patient is in shock, has pulmonary edema or has severe chest pain, he should receive immediate emergency care; otherwise, he should be admitted to the Medical Ward for treatment. Outlined below is the specific therapy for the respective dysrhythmias.
   b. It should be emphasized that *effective oxygen therapy* will always produce improvement in the patient with a cardiac dysrhythmia. Oxygen therapy can be given by face mask, nasal catheter, etc., and should continue as the patient is transported to a hospital bed.

6. **The Most Common Acute Dysrhythmias: The Tachycardias.**
   a. *Sinus tachycardia.* — Sinus tachycardia is not usually a serious dysrhythmia. It often is caused by fever, anxiety, hyperthyroidism, drugs, etc. The immediate treatment is sedation; further care depends on the underlying cause.
   b. *Paroxysmal Atrial Tachycardia.*
      1) In the absence of cardiac disease, most attacks of paroxysmal atrial tachycardia subside spontaneously.
      2) In this and any cardiac dysrhythmia, the Emergency physician is cautioned not to use therapeutic remedies that are more dangerous than the disease.
      3) **Treatment** consists of drug therapy and non-pharmacologic measures such as vagal stimulation, etc.
         a) *Nonpharmacologic measures.* — The patient is instructed to do the Valsalva maneuver. After a deep breath and while

holding his breath, the patient "bears down" by contracting his chest and abdominal muscles. Simultaneously, he stretches his arms and body and lowers his head between his knees.

b) *Vagal stimulation.*—With the patient relaxed, on his back, gentle but firm pressure and massage are applied to one carotid sinus for 10-20 seconds. One should not massage both carotid sinuses at the same time. During this maneuver, the cardiac rhythm should be observed.

c) Bilateral *pressure* over the eyeballs has been suggested. This method usually is ineffective, and it may produce retinal detachment or other damage to the eyes.

d) *Vomiting,* induced by digital stimulation of the pharynx by the patient may be effective.

e) A digitalis preparation.

c. *Nodal tachycardia.*

1) For this condition, the electrocardiogram is the diagnostic aid. Atrial P waves are inverted, the P-R interval is short and the QRS complexes are of normal configuration.

2) Digitalis and quinidine should be withheld unless congestive heart failure is present. If the patient is receiving digitalis preparations, they should be discontinued; the patient should be sedated and admitted to the hospital. Direct current synchronized countershock has been found useful.

d. *Atrial flutter.*

1) An atrial flutter is an infrequent dysrhythmia. The atria beat regularly at a rate of 250-300 per minute.

2) Digitalis is the drug of choice, with rapid digitalization using intravenous lanatoside C. If atrial fibrillation develops, quinidine therapy can be introduced. *Caution:* Quinidine

should not be given *before* digitalization, for
ventricular tachycardia may be precipitated.

   e. *Paroxysmal ventricular tachycardia.*

      1) If digitalis intoxication is suspected as a cause
of paroxysmal ventricular tachycardia, the
drug should be discontinued.

      2) Lidocaine, 75 mg., I.V. in bolus form can be
given initially, followed by a 2-3 mg./minute
infusion, if needed.

      3) I.V. pronestyl can also be used at a rate of
100 mg./minute but hypotension is a frequent
side effect. Direct-current synchronized
countershock offers an effective rapid measure of conversion.

   f. *Atrioventricular heart block—Stokes-Adams
syndrome.*

      1) I.V. atropine sulfate, 1 mg., should be used
to see if blockage of vagal tone will increase
the rate. This dose can be repeated every 4
hours.

      2) Isuprel infusion of 2 mg. in 200 ml. of 5%
D/W with constant monitoring at a rate of
0.5 ml. to 1 ml./minute to titrate an increase
in rate without PVC's.

      3) A transvenous cardiac pacemaker probably is
the most reliable method if the above two
drugs are ineffective.

7. *Irregular Dysrhythmias.*—The acute irregular dysrhythmias are the atrial, ventricular and flutter
fibrillations.

   a. *Atrial fibrillation.*

      1) This is the most common dysrhythmia. No
emergency treatment is necessary if the patient has a slow ventricular rate and is not in
acute distress.

      2) If the ventricular rate is rapid, the patient
should be intravenously digitalized with
cedilanid to slow the ventricular rate. If this
does not produce a normal sinus rhythm,

quinidine can be used. The patient should be hospitalized.

b. *Ventricular fibrillation.*

  1) This is an irregular dysrhythmia which is characterized by an ineffective ventricular contraction.

  2) The treatment is urgent, using direct-current countershock to the anterior thorax (see Fig. 14-1).

  3) Measures of heart-lung resuscitation with external cardiac compression similar to that of cardiac arrest are instituted.

c. *Flutter fibrillation.*

  1) Battery-operated electronic devices to monitor the electrocardiogram are also useful in the direct-current synchronized cardioversion

Fig. 14-1.—Portable battery-operated electrocardioscope, pacemaker, and direct current defibrillator. A synchronized countershock can be given to the chest through the hand-operated electrodes.

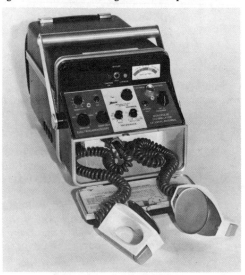

of the flutter fibrillation.

    2) Unless the cardioversion must be done as an emergency, the patient should be admitted to the hospital for elective cardioversion with direct-current synchronized counter-shock. Cardioversion should be used with extreme caution in the elderly patient.

D. ACUTE MYOCARDIAL INFARCTION

See Chapter 2, "Emergency Care of Acute Myocardial Infarction."

E. ACUTE PULMONARY EDEMA

1. Acute severe pulmonary edema constitutes a grave medical emergency. The patient with pulmonary edema is terrified because of sensations of suffocation and imminent death.

2. Treatment consists of placing the patient in the proper upright position, the use of drugs and oxygen, automatic rotating tourniquets and reduction of blood volume (see Fig. 14-2).

3. The patient should have his chest and head elevated and his feet in a dependent position.

4. Morphine sulphate, 15-30 mg., with atropine sulfate, 0.4 mg. s.c., can relieve anxiety and depress the pulmonary reflexes. Oxygen should be administered in high concentrations by tent or by a tight-fitting mask. Oxygen flow must exceed the patient's demand.

5. The blood volume can be reduced by external phlebotomy, 300-1000 ml. of blood can be withdrawn rapidly from the patient. Caution must be exercised to determine that the patient does not have an anemia.

6. Internal phlebotomy requires the use of soft rubber tourniquets to apply sufficient pressure to obstruct venous but not arterial blood flow. They are applied to three of the four extremities in rotation for 15-minute periods.

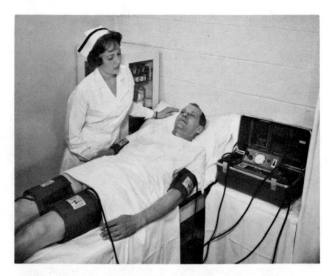

Fig. 14-2.—Automatic rotating tourniquets in the treatment of a patient with pulmonary edema. The tourniquet is inflated and deflated automatically every 11¼ minutes.

7. Automatic rotating tourniquets are most effective in producing and sustaining an internal phlebotomy. In addition, automatic tourniquet mechanisms have not only benefited the patient but also freed nursing personnel to attend other patients.
8. Aminophylline, 0.5 Gm. I.V., is given over a 5-minute period. Ethacrynic acid or Lasix can produce a rapid and effective diuresis.
9. Rapid digitalization is of great value. This can be obtained by giving lanatoside C, 0.8-1.6 mg. I.V. All patients with acute pulmonary edema should be admitted to the Intensive Treatment Unit.

VIII. MANAGEMENT OF PULMONARY DISORDERS

See Chapter 9, "Emergencies of the Respiratory System."

A. ACUTE PNEUMONIA

1. The diagnosis is usually made from the history of fever, cough, pleuritic chest pain and productive sputum.
2. Sputum and blood cultures, total leukocyte and differential counts are obtained.
3. A chest x-ray film is made as soon as possible. It may be necessary to start oxygen before the patient leaves the Emergency Service.

B. PULMONARY EMBOLISM

1. Emergency treatment of patients with acute circulatory collapse from massive pulmonary embolism is unsatisfactory.
2. Oxygen is given for dyspnea and cyanosis.
3. Vasodilator agents are used to combat shock.
4. Meperidine (Demerol) and atropine are given to relieve pain.
5. Intravenous heparin should be given until oral anticoagulants are effective. All patients with acute pulmonary embolism should be admitted to the hospital.
6. *Immediate surgery* may be lifesaving.

IX. MANAGEMENT OF GASTROINTESTINAL DISORDERS

A. ACUTE NONSURGICAL ABDOMEN (see Chap. 10)

1. The primary consideration in the evaluation of abdominal symptoms is to determine whether or not an early operation is necessary.
2. In general, *nonsurgical* disease is characterized by inconsistent physical findings. Pain, even though severe, shifts from place to place or is diffuse.
3. One must be aware that myocardial infarction can result in severe abdominal pain. The following is a *partial list of medical conditions which can give rise to signs or symptoms simulating an acute surgical abdomen.*

  a. *Abdominal viscera* (ulcerative colitis, regional ileitis, tablets containing potassium chloride, acute diverticulitis, acute hepatic porphyria, amebic hepatitis, pyogenic or amebic liver abscess, hepatoma, fecal impaction, rectal spasm, pain due to intestinal ischemia).

  b. *Kidneys* (acute pyelonephritis, nephrolithiasis, papillary necrosis, renal infarction).

  c. *Central nervous system* (abdominal migraine, epilepsy, tabes dorsalis, spinal cord tumors, herpes zoster).

  d. *Endocrine system* (diabetes mellitus, hyperthyroidism).

  e. *Blood* (sickle cell anemia, hemolytic crises).

  f. *Lungs* (basal pneumonia, diaphragmatic pleurisy).

  g. *Collagen diseases* (systemic lupus erythematosus, rheumatic fever, polyarteritis nodosa, Henoch's purpura).

  h. *Metabolic disturbances* (porphyria, essential hyperlipenia).

  i. *Poisonings* (methanol, ethanol, arsenic, lead, carbon tetrachloride).

  j. *Parasites* (amebiasis, ascariasis, strongyloidiasis, pinworms, etc.).

B. ACUTE GASTROENTERITIS (vomiting and cholera-like diarrhea)

 1. Acute "food poisoning" results from the ingestion of noxious agents or enterotoxins secreted by bacteria. Suspicion of food poisoning should arise when a patient presents with febrile gastroenteritis of acute onset, especially if more than one member of a family or group develops the same illness.

 2. Treatment consists of the following:

  a. Overcome dehydration and electrolyte imbalance by the use of dextrose-saline solutions with added supplements of potassium chloride.

  b. Observe for circulatory collapse.

    c. Obtain stool specimen for microscopic examination for ova and parasites and for specific bacteriologic cultures.

    d. Treat nausea with parenteral Compazine, 10 mg. I.M.

    e. Relieve intestinal tract cramps (atropine, 0.4 mg. and Demerol, 50 mg. I.M.).

X. MANAGEMENT OF EXPOSURE AND THERMAL INJURY

A. ELECTRIC SHOCK

1. Direct current is less dangerous than alternating current. Alternating current of high frequency or high voltage may be less dangerous than low-frequency or low-voltage current. *Ventricular fibrillation* may occur as the result of low-voltage alternating current. *Respiratory failure* may occur with high-voltage alternating current.

2. Heart-lung resuscitation is most important to sustain life until a direct-current countershock is delivered to the heart.

3. Many electric and telephone utility companies have given extensive training to their service men in the A-B-C's of heart-lung resuscitation. This has greatly aided in the survival of the electrically shocked person.

4. Electric shock may produce loss of consciousness. This may be brief or prolonged. After recovery from the initial shock, the patient may have complaints of muscle pain, fatigue, headache and nervous irritability. Electrical burns are usually sharply demarcated, round or oval areas. Tissue damage is usually severe.

5. The patient usually enters the Emergency Service in shock with pulmonary difficulties and, at times, with ventricular fibrillation.

6. Positive-pressure oxygen should be applied immediately to patients with respiratory paralysis. A

direct-current synchronized defibrillator, if available, can be used to correct the dysrhythmia.

7. Vasopressor agents can be given to correct the shock. *Care* should be taken in the administering of parenteral fluids to prevent pulmonary edema resulting from sudden congestive heart failure or internal hemorrhage. The initial treatment of electrical burns is similar to that of flame burns.

B. HEATSTROKE OR SUNSTROKE

1. Heatstroke is due to prolonged exposure to high temperatures or sun rays. It is characterized by sudden unconsciousness, hyperpyrexia and absence of sweating.
2. After the patient regains consciousness, there may be complaints of headache, dizziness, nausea and visual disturbances.
3. The skin is found to be flushed, hot and dry. The pulse is rapid and weak and temperature may be as high as 106°-110°F.
4. Emergency measures should be taken to reduce the high temperature.
   a. Remove the patient's clothing and cool him by fanning him after water is sprinkled on the body. Massage the extremities.
   b. Infuse normal saline solution slowly.
   c. Aspirin suppositories, 500 mg., can be given. Avoid sedation, as this further disturbs the heat-regulating mechanisms.
   d. If necessary, immerse the patient in cooled water. Use ice packs, a cold-water mattress or cold-water enemas.
   e. All patients with heatstroke should be admitted to the hospital. Check for acute *renal* failure and myoglobinuria.

C. HEAT EXHAUSTION

1. Following sustained exposure to heat, salt depletion and dehydration may occur. Subsequently, there is

a collapse of the peripheral circulation.

2. The patient complains of weakness, stupor, headache and dizziness. There may be muscle cramps.
3. Examination may reveal mental confusion and muscular incoordination, cool, pale skin and profuse perspiration, which may be associated with oliguria and tachycardia.
4. The patient should be placed in a cool place and his feet elevated. Infuse isotonic saline solution slowly, intravenously.
5. Shock should be treated if it occurs.
6. Should the patient have had excessive sweating and also ingested large quantities of sodium chloride, he may have hypokalemia. Check for acute renal failure and myoglobinuria.

D. COLD INJURY (FROSTBITE)

1. Patients with superficial frostbite complain of numbness, stinging and burning of the affected parts. With increased severity of freezing there may be parasthesias and stiffness.
2. As the frozen tissues thaw, the patient complains of burning pain and tenderness.
3. The skin may be white or yellow in color and there may be associated edema, blisters, necrosis and gangrene.
4. **Treatment.**
   a. Warm the patient with blankets and give soup, coffee, etc.
   b. Remove all covering from the injured parts.
   c. Thaw the injured part. Gradual rewarming with water or air of 90°-104° F. may have already been started.
   d. Recent experience indicates that *rapid REWARM-ING* in water of 110°-115° F. during a 20-minute period may be very advantageous. It is given at least twice daily.
   e. A whirlpool bath containing pHisoHex is ideal.
   f. An analgesic may be used if necessary.

g. The patient is isolated and strict aseptic precautions are observed. Prevention of infection is of extreme importance.

h. No dressings are used. Sterile sheets over the thorax and abdomen support the hand.

i. If the feet are injured, apply sterile cotton between the toes; no walking is permitted.

j. An exercise program of both upper and lower extremities is begun immediately. Each digit and joint is put through a full range of motion for 10 minutes each hour.

k. Give tetanus toxoid (see Chap. 7). If open lesions are present, antibiotics may be indicated (see Part I, 4).

l. Admit the patient to the hospital. Subsequent care may include sympathetic ganglion blocks, heparin or procaine.

m. Avoid bleb rupture, debridement or early amputation.

E. DECOMPRESSION SICKNESS

1. Too rapid decompression of compressed-air workers, underwater divers and aviation personnel may give rise to the formation of fine bubbles in the blood and fatty tissues.

2. These bubbles produce characteristic symptoms of joint, bone and muscle pain with paralysis (the bends) and asphyxia (the chokes).

3. Lesser symptoms of pruritus and skin rash occur if the skin is cooled during decompression.

4. The indication of bubbles in the lungs is the presence of substernal distress on deep inspiration. This frequently induces coughing, especially if smoking.

5. Treatment is as follows:

   a. Use immediate and prolonged recompression on all patients, no matter how mild the symptoms.

   b. Give oxygen therapy.

   c. Treat for shock.

6. Admit all patients to the hospital if a recompression chamber is present; otherwise, transfer to the nearest facility for definitive therapy.

CHAPTER 15

Obstetric and Gynecologic Emergencies

WILLIAM F. MENGERT, M.D.

I. INTRODUCTION

A. Correct diagnosis in obstetric and gynecologic emergencies depends on four basic factors:
   1. A good history.
   2. Knowledge.
   3. A high index of suspicion.
   4. Educated touch.

B. The usual reasons for a woman coming to the Emergency Service are:
   1. Abdominal pain.
   2. Vaginal bleeding.
   3. A combination of both.

C. *Every pregnant woman* coming to the Emergency Service must be seen by a specialist in Obstetrics and Gynecology, her personal physician, or both.

II. ABDOMINAL PAIN

A. If *lower quadrant pain* is present, consider:
   1. Ectopic pregnancy.
   2. Pyelonephritis of pregnancy (flank pain).
   3. Twisted cyst.
   4. Pelvic inflammatory disease.
   5. Appendicitis.
   6. Cystitis.

B. If *generalized pain* is present, consider:
1. Labor.
2. Abortion.
3. Ruptured viscus.
4. Peritonitis (there is always some peritonitis with an initial attack of pelvic inflammatory disease).
5. Tumor with accident, such as a twisted pedicle or infection.

III. VAGINAL BLEEDING

A. OBVIOUSLY PREGNANT

1. Placental abruption.
2. Placenta previa.
3. Labor.

B. NOT OBVIOUSLY PREGNANT

1. Abortion.
2. Advanced cervical cancer.
3. Adolescent menorrhagia.
4. Pelvic inflammatory disease (P.I.D.) in a late manifestation.

C. HYPOTENSION AND SHOCK

1. Abortion.
2. Second-trimester pregnancy bleeding.
3. Internal hemorrhage from *ectopic pregnancy*.
4. Late pregnancy postural hypotension.
    a. Can the patient *sit up*? If so, does the situation worsen or improve? Postural hypotension is the only one which improves.

D. MENSTRUAL ABERRATION.

1. Ectopic pregnancy. DOES NOT DEPEND ON A PERIOD OF AMENORRHEA for diagnosis. *Think of it always* when there is a change in menstrual habit.

      a. It must be considered seriously in first trimester pregnancy.

      b. The classic triad consists of:
          1) Menstrual disturbance.
          2) Vaginal bleeding.
          3) An adnexal mass.

      c. *Any* or *all* of these may not be found!

      d. A rapid pulse, hypotension and a low hematocrit must *alert* the physician to an ectopic pregnancy.

      e. Pelvic examination may reveal:
          1) Pain with motion of the cervix.
          2) An enlarged uterus.
          3) An adnexal mass, usually unilateral.

      f. Do *not* wait for results of a gravidex, or other test.

      g. Culdocentesis may be negative. Rely upon judgment!

      h. Begin I.V. fluids at once.

      i. Send blood for typing and cross-match.

      j. A hemorrhagic corpus luteum cyst must be considered.

  2. Idiopathic.

  3. Pelvic inflammatory disease.

      a. Ovarian tumors, except the dysontogenic group, do not change the menstrual pattern.

      b. Fibroid tumors do not cause amenorrhea.

E. Certain causes of bleeding in the *third trimester* can be *fatal* very rapidly. Expert consultation and treatment is needed *at once*.

IV. VULVAL MASS

A. A mass can be due to:
  1. Prolapsed genitalia.
  2. Abscess.
  3. Tumor.
  4. Small or large bowel hernia.

B. Expert consultation should be obtained if there is any doubt as to diagnosis and treatment.

V. ABDOMINAL MASS

A. May be due to:
1. Cyst.
2. Myoma.
3. Pelvic inflammatory disease.
4. Hematoma from an old ectopic pregnancy.
5. Abdominal pregnancy.

B. Small masses *tend to twist.* Large ones do not.

C. Differentiate a *large* cystic mass from ascites by palpation and percussion.

D. Do *not* use a trocar.

VI. CONVULSIONS

A. Eclampsia is characterized by:
1. Convulsions followed by coma.
2. Hypertension.
3. Edema.
4. Albuminuria.
5. Must be differentiated from epilepsy.

B. **Treatment**
1. Record vital signs, initially and regularly.
2. Send blood for:
    a. Type and cross-match.
    b. Complete blood count.
    c. Glucose level (especially if the patient is a diabetic).
3. Begin a salt-free infusion.
4. Insert a urinary bladder catheter to:
    a. Test for glucose and albumin.
    b. Monitor output.
5. Start a special flow-sheet—all medications, time given, vital signs, etc., must be recorded in an orderly fashion.
6. Give the patient moderate doses of the sedative of your choice. (There is NO known drug that will abort eclamptic convulsions.)

      a. During the convulsive-comatose stage, limit quantity of intravenous fluids to 2500 ml. per 24 hours in order to *avoid pulmonary edema.*

  7. Insert a padded tongue blade if needed.

VII. IMPORTANT DIFFERENTIAL DIAGNOSES

A. TRUE VERSUS FALSE LABOR

	True	False
1. Pain	a. Chiefly in back	Chiefly in abdomen
	b. Walking intensifies	Walking relieves
	c. Regular	Irregular
	d. Strength of contractions increases	Strength of contractions remains the same
	e. Frequency increases	Frequency remains the same
	f. Facial grimace	Facial muscles calm
2. Show	Often present	Seldom present
3. Membranes	Often ruptured	Seldom ruptured
4. Cervix	Effaced	Thick
	Dilating, 3 cm.+	Closed, not dilating

B. ECTOPIC PREGNANCY VERSUS PELVIC INFLAMMATORY DISEASE

(See Part I, 4)

	Ectopic	P.I.D.
1. Menses	Change in cycle, often absent	Normal or increased flow
2. Pain	Unilateral and seldom related to cycle	Coincident with period; usually bilateral, often becomes generalized
3. Syncope	Common	Rare
4. Vaginal discharge	Brownish to bloody, seldom excessive	Present in acute, not a factor in chronic
5. Tenderness	Mild, unilateral	Often bilateral
6. Mass	Unilateral	?
7. Temperature	Normal or slightly raised	Often elevated
8. Blood pressure	Unaffected or hypotension	Normal
9. Pulse	Elevated, if in *shock*	Elevated coincident with *fever*
10. Hematocrit	Normal or decreased	Normal
11. W.B.C.	Normal or slightly elevated	Normal or markedly elevated, 15,000+

12. Since P.I.D. and ectopic pregnancy are confused so frequently, if in any doubt, *hospitalize* the patient.

C. DIFFERENTIAL DIAGNOSIS

  1. **Acute P.I.D.**
     a. Vaginal discharge usual.
        1) Do gram-stain, take culture and sensitivities.
     b. Blood pressure usually normal.
     c. Pulse increase, if present, related to elevated temperature.
     d. Hematocrit stable.

    e.   W.B.C.—normal to significant increase.
    f.   Shock—uncommon (see ruptured abscess).
    g.   Signs of pregnancy usually absent.
    h.   No adnexal mass, as a rule.
    i.   Acute pain on motion of cervix.
    j.   If in any doubt, *admit.*

2. Appendicitis.

    a.   Typically, pain begins around umbilicus, then gravitates to right lower quadrant.
    b.   No relation to periods.
    c.   Nausea and vomiting often occur early.
    d.   Fever and elevated W.B.C. less evident than acute in P.I.D.
    e.   Point tenderness (McBurney's point) more common, *except* in retrocecal disease.

3. Diverticulitis.

    a.   More common in the elderly.
    b.   Often left-sided, but can be right-sided or bilateral.
    c.   Pelvic examination negative or equivocal.
    d.   Usually not pregnant.
    e.   Fever if rupture has occurred.
    f.   Rectal bleeding usually minimal or absent—may be massive.
    g.   Peritonitis if ruptured.
    h.   Barium enema diagnostic.

4. Chronic P.I.D.

    a.   History usually makes diagnosis.
    b.   Vaginal discharge:
        1) May be absent.
        2) Gram-stain often negative.
    c.   Tenderness usually bilateral.
    d.   Vital signs usually reliably reflect stage of infection.
    e.   If intestinal obstruction is present:
        1) Signs and symptoms present.
        2) Examination may make the diagnosis.
        3) Plain film of the abdomen very helpful—but must be interpreted with care.

5. **Rupture of Tubo-Ovarian Cysts.**
   a. If large, must be differentiated from ascites.
   b. Nausea is common, vomiting is rare.
   c. Use of a *trocar* or *large needle* is *contraindicated.*
   d. Rupture results in:
      1) An acutely ill patient.
      2) Signs and symptoms of acute peritonitis.
      3) Requires a thorough, rapid work-up and usually surgical intervention.
      4) Abscess is often present and must be treated with great care.

6. Almost *all drugs* cross the placenta and affect the fetus. Obtain consultation before giving *any* drug to a pregnant female.

VIII. THIRD TRIMESTER BLEEDING

A. Third trimester bleeding may be:
   1. Merely a heavy show signaling labor.
   2. Placenta previa or abruptio placentae.
      a. Both of these may be life-threatening to the mother if not managed well.
   3. All patients who bleed late in pregnancy *must* have the benefit of immediate obstetrical consultation in the Emergency Service.

B. *No vaginal or rectal examinations may be performed on a patient with third trimester bleeding in any circumstances.* If the patient has *placenta previa,* a vaginal or rectal examination may provoke torrential or fatal hemorrhage.

C. The responsibility of the Emergency Service physician is to call the obstetrical consultant immediately and prepare for emergency admission. He should draw blood for type cross-match and insert a large bore needle for intravenous transfusions.

D. The patient with painless, bright red bleeding in the third trimester must be considered to have placenta previa until proved otherwise.

E. The obstetrical consultant may elect to perform a gentle speculum examination to rule out local traumatic or neoplastic causes of the bleeding.

F. Digital examination may be performed *only* in the operating room with complete preparation for cesarean section.

G. Definitive diagnosis and mangement of placenta previa are exclusively inpatient procedures.

IX. ABRUPTIO PLACENTAE

A. This complication is classically characterized by vaginal bleeding in the third trimester, often with hypertonic, painful uterine contractions. Pain may be absent and bleeding may be concealed.

B. Fetal death, as witnessed by absence of fetal heart tones, may have occurred by the time the patient reaches the Emergency Service.

C. No attempts at definitive diagnosis should be made in the Emergency Service.

D. Obstetrical consultation should be called and the patient admitted.

E. Blood is drawn for typing and cross-matching and an intravenous infusion is started through a large-bore needle.
   1. The blood should be observed for *clotting,* for some cases of severe abruptio placentae are complicated by hypofibrinogenemia.
   2. *Renal tubular damage* may result in oliguria.

X. PREMATURE RUPTURE OF THE MEMBRANES

A. Any patient who complains of vaginal discharge must be seen by an obstetrical consultant.

B. If leakage of amniotic fluid from the vagina can be demonstrated, the patient is admitted.

C. Patients with intrauterine infection are delivered promptly.

XI. AMNIOTIC FLUID EMBOLISM

A. This complication is rare but very dangerous and usually occurs during or immediately after delivery.

B. It may be associated with persistent bleeding and the patient usually is dyspneic, cyanotic, in shock and may have pulmonary edema.

C. When severe, the patient rarely survives. Obstetrical consultation should be called immediately.

D. **Treatment**
   1. Oxygen and I.V. fluids at once.
   2. If a clotting defect is detectable, prompt treatment is required.

XII. CYSTITIS AND ACUTE PYELONEPHRITIS

A. These are very common complications of pregnancy.

B. The DIAGNOSIS is established by:
   1. History.
   2. Physical findings.
   3. Examination of a clean, voided specimen.

C. **Treatment**
   1. An obstetrician and urologist should work together to:
      a. Establish the diagnosis.
      b. Find the cause (obstruction, etc.) (see Chap. 16).
      c. Select the appropriate antimicrobials which will be effective yet *not* endanger the fetus.

XIII. PROCEDURE FOR SUSPECTED RAPE

A. *Be objective. Offer no opinions* as to whether or not you think the patient was raped. Each of these is a potential court case.

B. *Get a good history.* Write down *only what the patient said* in her own words.
   1. Did she fight back?
   2. Are her clothes torn?

C. *Examine* the woman, especially in the regions of the
    lower abdomen, buttocks and external genitalia for evi-
    dence of trauma.
    1. Look at introitus, including hymen.
    2. Make speculum examination of the cervix.
    3. Obtain hanging drop of vaginal pool from posterior
        vault, for sperm.
    4. Obtain a dried smear of same.
    5. Send clearly labeled smear to Pathology.
    6. Give no opinion.
    7. You may tell the police what you saw and found.
    8. Never say or write in the chart whether or not the
        patient was raped.

XIV. FOUR DO'S AND FOUR DON'TS

A. DO:

1. Speculum examination (gentle) in all bleeding
    women.
2. Remove obvious placental tissue from external cerv-
    ical os.
3. Prepare for possible transfusion in all women with
    obvious hemorrhage, by starting intravenous infu-
    sion, even if the patient is not bleeding.
4. THINK ALWAYS OF PREGNANCY, especially
    ECTOPIC.

B. DON'T:

1. Examine suspected abruptions and previas digitally
    either by vagina or rectum.
2. Plunge a trocar for diagnostic purposes into the ab-
    domen of a woman with obvious fluid.
3. Send a patient with pelvic inflammatory disease
    home on douches and antibiotics without a return
    appointment the next day to clinic. She may have
    an ectopic pregnancy.
4. Send *any* woman with obvious pregnancy or genital
    disease away from Emergency until a resident from
    Obstetrics and Gynecology or attending physician
    has seen her.

CHAPTER 16

Emergency Service Management of Genitourinary Problems

SAMUEL S. CLARK, M.D.C.M., V. SRINIVASAN, M.D., *and* JOSEPH H. KIEFER, M.D.

I. INTRODUCTION

A. Although serious urologic emergencies are not very common, increasing numbers of injuries to the urinary tract are seen with the rise in automobile and industrial accidents. The usual urologic emergencies seen in our Emergency Service are: acute urinary retention, hematuria, colic due to stones, upper and lower urinary tract infections, trauma to the kidney, trauma to the bladder and urethra in relation to bony pelvic trauma, trauma to penis and scrotum, acute testicular enlargement, priapism and paraphimosis. The majority of these conditions can be treated conservatively pending specific evaluation, but a few of them need emergency surgery.

B. An adequate and thorough history, physical examination and a few simple diagnostic aids, including roentgenograms, will usually localize the site and nature of pathology and aid in determining the need for immediate hospitalization.

II. GENITOURINARY TRACT INJURIES

A. RENAL INJURIES

1. The kidney is fortunately infrequently injured due to its mobility, its protection by heavy musculature and the rib cage and its retroperitoneal position.

Because of the soft nature of its parenchyma and
extreme vascularity, it cannot withstand severe blunt
or perforating injuries and is easily liable to undergo
laceration. Often, the fatty capsule of the kidney
acts as a safety valve by limiting the bleeding due to
pressure by the confined hematoma.

2. The injuries are more common in younger persons.
   The *types* of renal injuries include:
   a. Contusion.
   b. Tear of the capsule.
   c. Rupture of the parenchyma.
   d. Rupture of the capsule, parenchyma and collect-
      ing system.
   e. "Fracture" of the parenchyma.
   f. Pulping of the parenchyma.
   g. Tear of the pedicle.
   h. Contusion of the pedicle with thrombosis of
      renal artery and/or vein (Fig. 16-1). The severity
      of the injury may be minimal, moderate or
      severe.

3. *Simple contusions* are negligible or minimal injuries,
   requiring very little treatment. With *rupture of the
   parenchyma,* the injury becomes moderate or severe, depending on the extent of blood loss and the
   loss of functional renal parenchyma. Rupture of the
   renal pelvis may occur and result in urinary extravasation; this is more likely in a previously diseased
   kidney, such as in hydronephrosis, pyonephrosis,
   tumors or abscesses.

4. *Blunt trauma* to the abdomen produces renal injury
   by transmitting the impact in all directions, as in a
   fluid-filled bag, or by impinging the kidney against
   a solid structure such as vertebrae.

5. *Penetrating* injuries are often associated with other
   visceral injuries and thorough inspection of the
   wound of entry and exit is necessary to assess the
   possible extent of internal injuries.

6. The *symptomatology* includes flank pain and tenderness, hematuria, shock, a flank mass which may be
   expanding, and abdominal guarding or rigidity. The

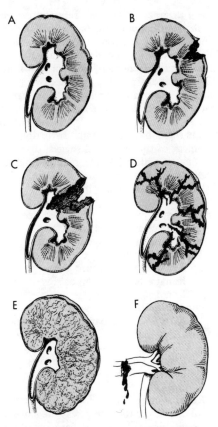

Fig. 16-1.—Renal injuries. A, tear of renal capsule. B, rupture of parenchyma. C, rupture of capsule, parenchyma, and pelvis. D, "fracture" of parenchyma. E, pulping of parenchyma. F, tear of renal pedicle.

patient may be in *shock,* to which attention should be directed.

7. Manage *the shock* before radiologic assessment. A

patient in shock will not excrete contrast medium and the resulting nonvisualization of the kidney may be mistaken for a seriously damaged kidney.

8. The full extent of renal damage may not be seen fully in an intravenous pyelogram (IVP); however, it helps to demonstrate the presence of a good functioning kidney on the *uninjured* side. Presence of at least a nephrogram on the injured side rules out renal arterial occlusion. Extravasation of the dye outside the collecting system, distortion, and displacement of the kidney all suggest urine and/or blood extravasation. Retrograde pyelography is usually unnecessary and may be harmful because of the risk of introducing infection.

9. An infusion pyelogram (1 ml./lb. body weight of contrast media) is recommended as a routine to demonstrate clearly the urinary tract.
    a. No visualization of dye indicates:
       1) Patient in shock.
       2) Renal arterial rupture.
       3) Renal arterial thrombosis.
       4) Renal vein damage.
    b. Poor visualization of dye indicates:
       1) All above, plus parenchymal damage.
    c. Visualization with extravasation and/or distortion indicates:
       1) Parenchymal and collecting system injury—hematoma, urinoma, urethral obstruction by clots.
    d. Renal angiography and aortography are very useful diagnostic tools to assess the state of renal vasculature and the need for arterial repair such as in renal artery contusion or tear.

10. **Treatment**
    a. In general, conservative measures are recommended, consisting of:
       1) Careful monitoring of vital signs and observation of size of flank mass.
       2) Recording urinary output and saving the voidings to compare the amount of blood.

This helps in assessing whether bleeding is
stopping or not.
3) Stabilizing blood pressure and pulse with
I.V. fluids and blood.
4) Repeating IVP, if necessary, after stabilizing
patient.
b. Surgery is indicated when the vital signs cannot
be maintained with adequate fluid and blood replacement, with an expanding flank mass, falling
central venous pressure (CVP) and continued
gross hematuria. However, in a stabilized patient,
with a stable flank mass, opening of Gerota's
fascia may restart the hemorrhage because of the
removal of the tamponade effect. Surgical exploration often results in nephrectomy and so
should be reserved for desperate cases.
c. Repair of parenchymal and collecting systems
and drainage of the perinephric space should be
attempted whenever possible. Partial nephrectomy is performed in injuries confined to either
pole. Surgical exploration is also indicated in all
penetrating abdominal injuries and, at the time
of celiotomy, primary repair of renal injury
should be done only if there is severe damage to
the parenchyma.

B. PERINEPHRIC ABSCESS

1. Bacteria may reach the perirenal tissues from distant
foci by the vascular or the lymphatic routes, by con-
tiguity or by extension. The renal lesions most frequently associated with perinephric abscess are calculus, renal abscess, pyonephrosis, rupture of the
collecting system and tuberculosis.
2. Lesions of the upper lumbar vertebrae, pancreatic
abscess and duodenal and appendicular perforations
posteriorly may lead to secondary perirenal abscess.
The occurrence of perinephric abscess secondary to
staphylococcus infections elsewhere (furuncles, carbuncles, etc.) is common enough to warrant thorough
inquiry when suspicion of such a lesion exists.

3. The *diagnosis* of a typical perinephric abscess is suspected in the presence of extreme costovertebral-angle tenderness, flank-muscle rigidity, flank mass and septic fever with chills.

4. X-ray evidence includes: renal area mass, displacement of the kidney, obliteration of psoas shadow and/or kidney outlines and curvature of the lumbar spine toward the affected side. Because of fixity of the kidney due to inflammation, the affected kidney does not move with respiration and can be detected if an IVP is taken with the patient breathing. *Surgical drainage* of the perirenal abscess and appropriate *antibacterial* medication is indicated without delay.

C. RENAL COLIC

1. Renal or ureteral colic is due to the passage of a stone through the ureter causing stretching of smooth muscle and hyperperistalsis above the site of the stone.

2. The *pain* is severe, radiating from flank to groin, often accompanied by nausea and/or vomiting and may be associated with microscopic hematuria. Since ureteral peristalsis is not known to be due to any specific innervation, anticholinergics which have been traditionally employed have no real scientific basis.

3. Pain is relieved by adequate sedation with narcotics. The patient is kept at rest and hydrated. The urine is strained for any calculus.

4. Emergency IVP's are becoming increasingly popular as an obstructed, dilated collecting system in the presence of infection and fever will need more drastic measures. A ureteral catheter is passed above the stone to relieve pain and fever and the patient is examined further.

D. URETERAL INJURIES

1. Injury of the ureter is rarely seen as a result of external trauma because of its well-protected position

and mobility. The most common cause is iatrogenic
due to instrumentation. This may cause an increasing mass in the flank or an increasing amount of free
fluid within the peritoneal cavity. Intravenous
urography may reveal the site of rupture and extravasation and frequently dilatation of the collecting
system above.

2. If visualization of the kidney fails, a retrograde pyelogram helps to delineate the site of injury, though
there is a potential risk of infection. Occasionally,
one may be successful in inserting a ureteral catheter above the site of injury which helps in drainage
as well as aids in surgery.

3. **Treatment** consists of drainage of the extravasated
urine with a nephrostomy to divert the flow of
urine. A stricture of the ureter may result, needing
elective repair at a later date.

E. BLADDER INJURIES

1. Rarely does the bladder rupture spontaneously. The
most common bladder injuries are perforation, tears
or avulsion either due to direct trauma or associated
with fractures of the bony pelvis. A distended bladder may suffer extensive injury from minimum
trauma, while an empty, collapsed bladder escapes.
Rupture of the bladder may be intra- or extraperi-
toneal.

2. The *treatment* of bladder perforation is *emergent*
and *never conservative*. The delay in treatment of
only a few hours leads to a marked increase in mortality, especially with intraperitoneal rupture of the
bladder.

3. The patient presents with the *history* of trauma, associated pelvic fractures, inability to urinate and
pain and rigidity in the suprapubic region.

4. An intravenous urogram reveals extravasated dye.
Classically, it is taught that a catheter should be inserted to see if any urine is obtained and, if only
blood or a small amount of blood-stained urine is
obtained, it is diagnostic of bladder perforation.

There is *risk of infection* in this method. Rectal examination will reveal a baggy fullness with loss of normal landmarks such as the prostatic outline.

5. A retrograde cystogram may be performed to delineate perforation if the urethra is shown to be intact by retrograde urethrogram.

6. *Exploration* is essential and drainage of the bladder by a suprapubic cystostomy tube and drainage of the perivesical space is mandatory.

F. URETHRAL INJURIES

1. *Posterior* urethral injuries (membranous and prostatic urethral) are classical accompaniments of *pelvic fractures. Anterior* urethral injuries follow *direct trauma* such as falling astride on the perineum ("straddle" injuries). Iatrogenic injuries due to instrumentation are frequent.

2. The anatomic division in extravasation from urethral perforation is the urogenital diaphragm. Injuries of the membranous and prostatic urethra allow extravasation superior to the urogenital diaphragm and along the periprostatic and perivesical fascial planes. Perforation of the urethra below the urogenital diaphragm permits extravasation into the superficial perineal space, scrotum and lower anterior abdominal wall.

3. Perforation of the bulbous and pendulous urethra similarly extravasates through the corpus spongiosum beneath and through Buck's fascia, beneath Colles' fascia of the perineum, the dartos muscle of the scrotum and penis and Scarpa's fascia of the anterior abdominal wall.

4. Extravasation laterally is restricted by attachments of the fascial elements to Poupart's ligament and below by the urogenital diaphragm.

5. Early in urethral injury *below* the urogenital diaphragm, *symptoms* may be so mild as to completely mislead the examiner; slight urethral bleeding, little pain and minimal perineal or scrotal swelling may

comprise the entire presenting picture. However, within a few hours following injury, the picture becomes one of constant local pain, difficulty or inability to urinate, a perineal or scrotal mass which may be fluctuant or woody-hard and pitting edema of the perineal and scrotal skin, leaving no doubt as to the lesion and organ involved.

6. *Diagnosis* of the site of rupture is established by a retrograde urethrogram performed under aseptic conditions. Introduction of a catheter as a diagnostic test is prone to the risk of infection and must be avoided.

7. A *simple suprapubic cystostomy* is done to divert urine and the hematoma is allowed to resolve spontaneously. Since urethral stricture is an inevitable sequelae of these injuries, immediate reapproximation of the urethral ends, though popular, is viewed with disfavor. It is much more preferable to do an elective repair at a later date.

G. URINARY RETENTION

1. Acute urinary retention may occur secondary to benign hyperplasia or carcinoma of the prostate, urethral stricture, acute prostatic infection, vesical or urethral calculus, hemorrhage and blood clot formation within the bladder or neurogenic disturbances of the bladder.

2. Immediate relief is achieved by inserting an indwelling Foley-type catheter. This may not be possible in patients who are in retention due to urethral strictures. In such cases, the stricture is dilated by a filiforms and follower bougies after which a catheter may be inserted. This must be done by a urologist.

3. The bladder is decompressed slowly to prevent bleeding by using initially a screw-clamp type arrangement and allowing urine to drip at a constant speed; later, a straight drainage bag is used. Clamping the catheter is not recommended as one may forget to remove the clamp.

4. If a catheter cannot be introduced, a suprapubic cystostomy is performed. If the urinary retention is due to blood clots, a large bore catheter is inserted to irrigate the clots with a Toomey or bulb syringe. Occasionally, a solid-wall tube, such as a cystoscope or resectoscope sheath, is necessary to evacuate the clots. It is essential to remove the clots, for not only does this relieve retention but, often, when the clots have been removed, the bladder contracts and bleeding practically ceases. If the clots cannot be evacuated by these methods, cystostomy may be required.

H. PENILE TRAUMA

1. Contusions of the penis are characterized by edema or in more serious injuries, by ecchymosis which spreads to the scrotum and even to the anterior abdominal wall. The treatment is rest, pressure dressing, ice packs, and indwelling urethral catheter if there is interference with urination.

2. *Fracture* of the penis results from severe trauma to the erect organ with resulting rupture of the corpora cavernosa. Bleeding into the subcutaneous tissues is extensive, with severe swelling and pain along the penile shaft. *Treatment* consists of evacuation of clots, hemostasis and anatomic repair of the ruptured fascia. When the sheath of the corpus cavernosum is torn, healing may result in scar formation with curvature of the erect penis. Accurate surgical repair will reduce these sequelae.

3. *Wounds* of the penis are rare, usually being gunshot, stab or razor wounds. Occasionally, avulsion occurs when clothing is caught in machinery.

4. **Treatment** is directed toward re-establishing continuity of the urethra, arrest of hemorrhage, saving of all viable tissues, anatomic reconstruction of the penis and prevention of secondary infection.

I. PARAPHIMOSIS

1. Paraphimosis is the result of retraction of a tight
    prepucial skin behind the glans penis which cannot
    be pulled forward to cover the glans. It is frequent-
    ly a result of masturbation. Failure to bring the
    skin forward immediately results in edema of the
    glans owing to the tight band of constriction that is
    formed by the prepuce at the coronal sulcus.
2. The patient *presents* with pain, edematous prepuce
    and glans, and a tight ring at corona. The immediate
    treatment consists of manual reduction of the pre-
    puce (Fig. 16-2). The thumbs are placed on the glans
    with the index and middle fingers of each hand be-
    hind the point of constriction and, as the glans is
    pushed backwards, the skin is pulled forward until
    completely reduced.
3. If edema is excessive, this type of reduction may be
    impossible. The edema could be reduced by multi-
    ple sterile needle punctures and wrapping with an
    elastic bandage for a few minutes. In some cases,
    the constricting band may have to be divided. After
    these maneuvers, the prepuce can usually be pulled

Fig. 16-2.–Manual reduction for paraphimosis.

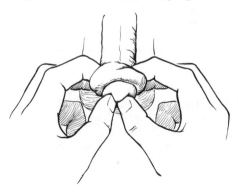

forward. Definitive treatment consists of elective circumcision at a later date.

J. INJURY OF SCROTUM AND ITS CONTENTS

1. The scrotum is commonly injured by kicks, blows, straddle-type injuries, during the playing of ball games, gunshot wounds, farm machinery accidents and in psychiatric patients' self-mutilation. Because of the extreme mobility of scrotal skin over its contents and because of the cremasteric action, the testes are somewhat less liable to trauma. However, when injured, a severe degree of testicular swelling due to traumatic orchitis, hydrocele or, more commonly, hematocele does occur. If the testes prolapse through an injury in the scrotal sac, they can be replaced and the laceration sutured.

2. Closed injuries of the scrotum and its contents are generally treated conservatively. A scrotal support is a must and when the patient is at rest, an adhesive tape may be placed across the thighs to be used as the support of the scrotum thus preventing further swelling of the loose tissues of the scrotum. Ice packs and analgesics are used along with the scrotal support. After 48 hours, warm, moist packs may be used. Occasionally, evacuation of the hematocele may be necessary.

3. Lacerations of the scrotum are treated by thorough cleansing, debridement and suturing of edges together with adequate drainage, if needed. Scrotal skin has a good blood supply and usually heals very well.

K. TORSION OF THE SPERMATIC CORD

1. Torsion of the spermatic cord, more frequently called torsion of the testes, is a twisting of the spermatic cord resulting in constriction of the blood supply and, if untreated, results in testicular atrophy. It is more common in children and young adults and in undescended testes.

2. The patient *presents* with acute onset of pain and scrotal swelling, sometimes nausea, vomiting and fever. This should be differentiated from acute epididymo-orchitis by the following signs: absence of signs of inflammation in the skin, no relief of pain on elevating the testis, shortening of the spermatic cord and raised position of the testis, firm tender testis, absence of signs of urinary infection on urinalysis and previous history of such episode spontaneously resolved. It should also be differentiated from strangulated hernia and testicular tumor.

3. Treatment consists of prompt surgical intervention on suspicion of the diagnosis of torsion. The testis is untwisted and anchored to the parietal layers of the scrotum. Because of the risk of torsion on the opposite side, usually orchiopexy is done on the contralateral side simultaneously.

L. ACUTE EPIDIDYMITIS

1. Acute nonspecific epididymitis is a common occurrence, usually secondary to lower urinary tract infection. Occasionally, the prime source of infection may be a septic focus elsewhere in the body.

2. The condition is usually unilateral with marked scrotal swelling, pain, heat, tenderness and redness and warmth of skin. The testis is frequently involved along with the epididymis and is enlarged and tender. This condition should be differentiated from torsion.

3. **Treatment** consists of elevation of scrotum with a scrotal support, antibiotics, analgesics and oral enzyme therapy. No instrumentation should be performed during acute episode, and after the subsidence of infection, primary urinary tract pathology is evaluated. A *urine culture* is indicated.

M. ANURIA

1. Occasionally, a patient may present with a history of not having urinated for several hours and in no

distress. The bladder will not be distended and catheterization may yield no urine. If there is any past history of renal disease, one may think in terms of renal failure. However, always to be ruled out is bilateral ureteral obstruction due to any cause (stones, retroperitoneal fibrosis, tumors, etc.).

2. The Emergency Service management consists of catheterizing the bladder, obtaining an intravenous urogram to see if the kidneys can be visualized and obtaining blood chemistries. If the IVP shows no visualization, urologic consultation should be sought to obtain retrograde pyelograms to rule out obstruction.

III. URINARY TRACT INFECTIONS

A. ACUTE CYSTITIS

Cystitis is more common in females. The presenting symptoms include frequency, urgency, dysuria, hematuria, suprapubic discomfort and sometimes backache. Urinalysis shows red and white blood cells and, possibly, bacteria. After a specimen is obtained for culture, the patient is treated with sulfisoxazole, nitrofurantoin, or nalidixic acid, and analgesics.

B. PROSTATITIS

1. Acute prostatitis is manifested by frequency, burning on urination, terminal hematuria, perineal discomfort or low backache and urethral discharge.

2. Rectal examination reveals a soft, boggy and tender prostate which may be enlarged. The prostatic fluid expressed after massage shows several white cells and/or bacteria. *Culture* of the prostatic fluid or postmassage urine may yield gram-negative organisms, though often no growth is obtained.

3. Treatment consists of antibiotics such as tetracycline or doxycycline, ampicillin, nitrofurantoin and analgesics. The patient is referred to the urology service for further evaluation.

C. ACUTE PYELONEPHRITIS

The patient *presents* with flank pain, fever, chills, hematuria, pyuria, frequency and occasionally burning. Costovertebral-angle tenderness, sometimes a palpable, tender kidney and white cells in the urine are diagnostic. It is essential to rule out obstruction (such as a stone in a ureter) as a cause of the pyelonephritis. This type of patient often needs hospitalization.

CHAPTER 17

Emergency Treatment of Convulsive Disorders

OSCAR SUGAR, M.D.

I. GENERAL CONSIDERATIONS

A. The major circumstances under which a patient may appear in the Emergency Room with convulsive disorders are (1) in a postictal state having had a seizure or (2) while having a seizure or series of seizures.

B. The neurologic disturbances following a seizure may range from a slight state of confusion to stupor, hemiparesis or hemiplegia or coma. If there is coma, *airway* must be ensured, blood drawn and lumbar puncture done to investigate the chief causes of coma.

II. PREVIOUS SEIZURES

A. If there is clear history of earlier seizures or if the patient bears identification as an epileptic, inquiry should be made as to type of medication used, doses missed, etc., and missing medication should be administered.

B. If the seizure has occurred in spite of regular medication, an extra dose of each medication may be given and the patient returned to the care of his regular physician. If such information is not available, or if there has been no prior treatment, the patient may be given 100 mg. phenobarbital by mouth or intramuscularly and sent home with an additional dose of medication to be taken in 4-6 hours, and with instruction to return promptly to his physician. The patient must be accompanied by a friend or relative.

C. If there is no personal physician, the patient may be referred to a staff neurologist or one of the neurology clinics in the city. He should, however, be observed for an hour to ensure the absence of further seizures which might incapacitate the patient or result in his prompt return. If the patient is found to have a persisting neurologic deficit or papilledema and has not had care for seizures or neurologic disease before, emergency hospitalization for investigation is warranted.

III. INFANTILE SEIZURES OR SPASM (HYPSARHYTHMIA)

These peculiar lightning-like jerks and bowing of the head, with pallor or cyanosis, crying and lack of attention may recur many times a day. They are usually found in postnatal infants, and are resistant to most forms of medication.

A. Phenobarbital sodium (3-5 mg./kg.) may be given slowly intravenously or by intramuscular injection to try to stop the immediate attack. The best available treatment is ACTH, which should be given intravenously *in the hospital.*

B. If phenobarbital does not stop the immediate attack, diazepam (Valium) may be given intravenously slowly in doses of up to 5 mg. (0.25 mg./kg., 1 mg./minute). In addition, paraldehyde (0.3 mg./kg.) mixed with an equal amount of mineral oil is given by rectal tube. If there is no depression of respiration and if tendon reflexes and pupils remain reactive, phenobarbital may be repeated every 60 minutes if necessary.

IV. STATUS EPILEPTICUS IN CHILDHOOD

A. The dose of phenobarbital to be given to children may be calculated on the basis of body weight (3-5 mg./kg., I.V. or I.M.) or body surface (125 mg./M^2 I.M. or I.V.).

B. Diazepam is more often the first medication: 0.4 mg./kg. up to a dose of 5-10 mg. would be proper.

C. Dilantin (diphenylhydantoin) is given in doses of 3-8 mg./kg./24 hours or 250 mg./M^2/24 hours.

V. STATUS EPILEPTICUS IN ADULTS

A. Intravenous diazepam is given slowly (no more than 1 mg. every 60 seconds) until 10-20 mg. is given or until respiratory depression is noted. Additional diazepam may be given intravenously over the next 12 hours (100 mg. in 500 ml. of 5% dextrose in lactated Ringer's or similar electrolyte solution).

B. If seizures persist, sodium amytal (sodium amobarbital) can be given slowly (500 mg. in 10-ml. solution, at a rate of 1 ml. or 50 mg. per minute). If the seizure stops, the medication should be stopped. Respiratory slowing is the important hazard.

C. Dilantin sodium (diphenylhydantoin) may be given at the same rate (50 mg./minute) for up to 500 mg. if necessary. Since this drug also affects the conducting system of the heart, care is needed if there is history of cardiac disturbance.

D. In addition, paraldehyde may be given slowly intravenously in doses of 3-5 Gm. If intramuscular use is contemplated, the injection should be deep in the muscle to avoid sterile abscess formation. Rectal paraldehyde (8-10 Gm. mixed with an equal volume of mineral oil) may be a useful adjunct, especially if veins are not available—but its action is delayed.

E. If barbiturates or diazepam are successful in stopping the seizure, diphenylhydantoin (Dilantin) may be started for more permanent control (250 mg. I.M. to be followed by 100 mg. q.i.d.).

F. In rare instances, it may be necessary (if seizures still continue) to request general anesthesia to stop the seizures; in an extreme case, the patient can be intubated paralyzed with succinylcholine, and put on a respirator.

G. Every patient who has been in status epilepticus should be hospitalized after controlling the initial seizure, because of the danger of respiratory depression, aspiration, prolonged sedation and immobility and repetition of seizures.

CHAPTER 18

Bone and Joint Trauma

RICHARD L. JACOBS, M.D.

I. INITIAL MEASURES

A. PRIORITIES

1. A system of priorities of treatment must be established for any patient with multiple injuries. An *adequate airway* must be established and maintained and gross *hemorrhage* controlled.
2. While *vital signs* are checked and recorded, intravenous infusion should be started and blood drawn for type and cross-match. If shock is present, plasma or a plasma expander may be used until whole blood is available.
3. Injuries to the *chest, abdomen* or *great vessels* require priority treatment since they may be critical.
4. If musculoskeletal injuries are found, appropriate *splints* must be applied before moving the patient. This helps prevent further injury and alleviates shock.
5. *Pain* should be relieved as soon as possible. In the absence of head injuries, appropriate analgesics may be used. If the patient has been in *shock* such medication should be given *slowly and intravenously*.
6. Substantial relief of *pain* will follow treatment and immobilization of the specific injury.
7. *Tetanus prophylaxis* must not be forgotten.
8. Any grossly apparent *musculoskeletal injury* requires an understanding of the mechanism of the injury. Check for possible *associated injuries* which may not be so apparent.

    a. Sciatic nerve injury in posterior dislocation of the hip.
    b. Spine injury in os calcis fractures.
    c. Kidney, spleen or liver injury in trauma to the torso are examples.

II. GENERAL CONSIDERATIONS

A. *Adequate roentgenograms* of the area of injury are imperative.
1. Postero-anterior, lateral and oblique views must be obtained.
2. Additional special views may be needed, such as "mortise" or oblique views in ankle injuries.
3. In *extremity* injuries, the *opposite side* is available as a control if you have any question as to interpretation of the film.
4. *Obtain comparison films, especially in children.*

B. *Early consultation* for treatment of associated *soft tissue* injuries may take lifesaving priority.
1. Do not assume sole responsibility for care of an injury which lies outside the area of your training or competence!
2. Most courts no longer apply the standard of local medical care in malpractice suits.
3. Your treatment of the patient *must be equal* to that given anywhere.

C. Anticipate the patient's needs in an orderly fashion.
1. Call for consultants in *advance* of need.
2. If surgery is necessary, alert the anesthetist and operating room staff as soon as possible.
3. The *radiology* departments should be notified of the need for x-ray control in the operating room.
4. Special instruments should be requested early. This should *never* be a cause for delay during the operation.

D. Open fractures should be debrided and thoroughly irrigated in the Main Operating Suite.
1. Clean wounds, not open longer than 6-8 hours, often

may be closed primarily (in civilian practice).
2. Gas gangrene still occurs after open fractures! Gram stain, cultures and sensitivities are indicated.
3. Be alert for *signs and symptoms* of this disastrous complication.
   a. Listlessness and diaphoresis.
   b. Increased fever, swelling, pain and a foul-smelling odor from the wound exudate.
   c. *Early radical* treatment may avoid amputation.
   d. *Hyperbaric oxygen* may be indicated.

E. Preservation of function is the primary consideration.
   1. Conservative treatment usually is indicated.
   2. A fracture of the distal third of the forearm in a child is best left in bayonet apposition, *not* anatomically reduced.
   3. An anatomic reduction of other fractures, such as ankle and hip, is indicated.
   4. In each instance, the treatment giving the *best functional result* with the least morbidity and mortality is conservative.

F. *Delayed union* due to:
   1. Loss of fracture hematoma.
   2. Loss of blood supply from surgical exposure.
   3. Wound infection after surgery must always be carefully considered.

G. **CASTS**

   1. An excessively padded and plaster cast is less comfortable and provides less immobilization than a *lightly* padded cast which is *well molded* to the contours of the limb.
   2. Plaster should not be dipped in warm water.
   3. Water at room temperature will allow time for adequate rubbing and contouring before the cast hardens.
   4. If the cast must later be split and spread, the padding must be divided *down to the skin,* otherwise underlying strands of sheet wadding may remain to impair circulation.

5. To prevent "window edema" of the soft tissues through cuts in the cast, fill the gap with fresh sheet wadding loosely held in place with an elastic bandage.

6. If a patient is not hospitalized after any cast is applied, be *certain* that he returns immediately if the extremity becomes cold, numb or if there is increased pain.

7. Examination the *next morning* may be too late.

8. For medico-legal protection, these instructions must be *written in the patient's record*.

9. Make a *drawing* of the injury on the cast.
   a. Indicate the *date* of the injury, of cast application and whether the injury was closed or open.

H. Roentgenograms (without removal of immobilization) should be obtained of any fracture or dislocation at 3 and at 10 days. If position is unsatisfactory, it can still be corrected.

I. Swelling and muscle weakness are often present after removal of a cast, especially in the lower extremities.
   1. This can be minimized by early care.
   2. After application of a well-molded cast, a patient can commence hourly isometric exercises with little or no pain to minimize muscle atrophy.
   3. Immediately after a cast is *removed* from a lower extremity, apply an *Unna boot* from toes to knee for about 10 days.
   4. This will help control swelling better than an elastic bandage.

J. *Records* must be *precise* and *complete*.
   1. They should contain nothing that would be inappropriate in court.
   2. Good medical treatment, well-documented, speaks for itself.
   3. *All instructions* to the *patient* must be *recorded* in detail in the chart.

K. *Overnight hospitalization* for close observation may be wise after apparently minor injuries. If there is any question, *admit* the patient.

L. Blanket operative permits are worthless. Even well-detailed permits have come under question in cases where it was claimed that the patient did not properly understand the terminology.

M. *Postreduction x-ray films* must *always* be made!

III. INJURIES OF THE UPPER EXTREMITY

A. CLAVICLE

Nonunion of fractures of the clavicle is uncommon. Hospitalization is necessary if there is marked displacement or neurovascular injury.

1. A sling may relieve much of the pain of undisplaced fractures. An active person will be more comfortable in a clavicular "T" splint.
2. This is fabricated by placing interlaced plaster splints on the patient's back with the horizontal arm of the T posterior to the scapulae (about 10 thicknesses of plaster). The vertical arm extends down over the *sacrum*.
3. After the splint has hardened, it is held in place by a 6-inch elastic bandage around the pelvis and vertical arm.
4. A 4-inch bandage around the shoulders in a figure-of-eight crossing posteriorly is then applied. The shoulders should be drawn back against the T. Simple figure-of-eight bandages without the T often fail to relieve discomfort and pain.
5. *If cosmesis* is a problem (as in a young girl wishing to avoid the appearance of a large mass of callus), complete bedrest on the back, with a sandbag between the shoulders may be elected.

B. SCAPULA

1. Fractures may be due to direct trauma or avulsion of muscle origins or insertions.
2. The patient should be examined closely for other associated injuries.

3. For simple fractures and most avulsions, sling immobilization during the period of the acute pain will be sufficient.

C. DISLOCATION OF THE SHOULDER

1. Dislocation is usually anterior and is quite apparent clinically. The lateral aspect of the shoulder is flat instead of rounded, and a deep sulcus is palpable between the head of the humerus and the acromion laterally.
2. Examination for associated *brachial plexus* injury is *mandatory*!
   a. Injury to the axillary nerve is common.
   b. It may be impossible to check for motor nerve injury to the deltoid because of pain, but hypesthesia indicates some compromise of sensory branches.
3. Record all your findings *before* reduction is attempted.
4. Have *adequate roentgenograms* to demonstrate any associated fractures.
5. The dislocation often can be reduced without active manipulation.
   a. The patient is given an appropriate dose of meperidine or morphine.
   b. He then lies face down on the examining table with shoulder over the edge and the affected extremity dependent.
   c. Ten to 15 pounds of weight is tied to the wrist with gauze bandages.
   d. The dislocation may reduce after 10-15 minutes of this traction.
   e. Manipulation under general anesthesia may be needed.
   f. If the patient has recently eaten or his physical condition prevents general anesthesia, injection of 5 ml. of 1% lidocaine into the shoulder joint usually will give adequate anesthesia.

6. **Method of Hippocrates.**
   a. Place your stockinged foot in the patient's axilla.
   b. Holding his wrist, exert slow, gentle longitudinal traction on the extremity.
   c. Then, slowly and without force, bring the extremity to the midline while maintaining traction.
7. **Kocher Maneuver.**
   a. This method has fallen into discredit because it has not been used properly.
   b. The patient's elbow is flexed acutely and longitudinal traction is exerted on the upper arm toward the foot of the table.
   c. While maintaining the traction, the shoulder is externally rotated and the elbow brought to the midline of the body.
   d. At this point, reduction should have been achieved.
   e. With *no force whatsoever,* the shoulder is then internally rotated and the palm placed on the opposite side of the chest, prior to immobilization.
   f. Iatrogenic injury occurs only when forceable internal rotation is attempted *before* reduction has been achieved.
8. After reduction of the dislocation by whatever means, it is the usual practice to immobilize the extremity by application of a swath (Velpeau) dressing with the arm on the chest.
   a. Bias-cut stockinette is good for this purpose.
   b. If the dressing tends to shift or become unwrapped, it may be covered with 1 roll of 6-inch plaster of paris bandage.
   c. Such a dressing is not rigid and will soften and crack, but the purpose is served (Fig. 18-1).
   d. Three weeks of immobilization will allow sufficient soft tissue healing to lessen chances of recurrent dislocation later.
   e. *Always* obtain postreduction films!

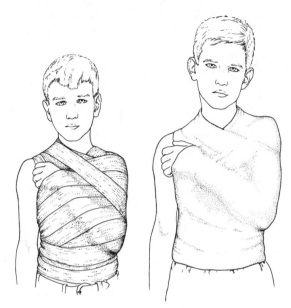

Fig. 18-1. —Swath (Velpeau) bandage.

D. **ROTATOR CUFF DISEASE** (supraspinatus tendonitis, subacromial bursitis)

1. The patient may complain of an acute onset of pain with motion of the shoulder.
2. The pain is unrelated to trauma and characteristically present only in the midrange of abduction, *not* with the arm at the side or with the arm fully elevated.
3. The pain is localized directly at the insertion of the supraspinatus muscle into the greater tubercle just inferior to the tip of the acromion.
4. There is not pain on pressure in this area with the arm elevated, as the tendon insertion then lies beneath the acromion and posteriorly.
5. In cases of a *tear* in the rotator cuff, the patient

may be unable to fully elevate the shoulder.

6. The disease process is due to degeneration of the rotator cuff, especially at the fibrous insertion of the supraspinatus.

7. The inflammatory process involves the overlying bursa, and is sometimes called subdeltoid or subacromial bursitis.

8. Calcium deposition may occur in the region of the insertion and is sometimes seen on x-ray film as a linear deposition extending medially from the tubercle and under the acromion.

9. Arthrography is not done frequently, but may demonstrate a tear in the rotator cuff.

10. Injection of 5 ml. of lidocaine and 10 mg. of hydrocortisone directly into the painful area usually will give immediate relief.

11. A sling should be applied and the patient warned that his pain probably will return and may even be increased when the effects of the lidocaine are gone (2-3 hours).

12. He should be given an analgesic and advised to apply *ice packs* to the shoulder if needed; *heat* should never be applied.

13. Symptoms should diminish in 2 or 3 days.

14. Large calcium deposits may be dealt with by "needling" or by 2-needle irrigation under local anesthetic. Surgical removal by a small deltoid-splitting incision sometimes is necessary.

15. Most cases respond well to conservative measures, but repeated injections of hydrocortisone (or any other steroid) into any joint should be *avoided.*

E. ACROMIOCLAVICULAR SEPARATION

1. The patient complains of pain localized at and just medial to the acromioclavicular joint.

2. The injury may involve torn ligaments of the joint only or, in more severe injuries, a tear of the coracoclavicular ligaments also—a complete acromioclavicular separation.

3. In the second instance, there will be much more prominence of the *upwardly displaced* distal end of the clavicle.

4. The only finding on examination may be local tenderness, but roentgenograms of the acromioclavicular joint (after injection of local anesthetic) with the patient holding about 10 pounds of weight in his hand on the injured side should readily demonstrate disruption of the joint.

5. Either injury may be treated conservatively.
   a. Circumferential strapping extending around the flexed elbow, up over the angle of the shoulder and the clavicle, may be used to hold the separation reduced.
   b. This is difficult to maintain. Frequent visits will be necessary to tighten the strapping.
   c. The patient may have complaints related to pressure upon the brachial plexus.

6. A *better* method is to place the extremity in a "military salute" position either with a shoulder spica or a manufactured splint which is left in place for 6-8 weeks.

7. It sometimes is elected, in complete separation, to hold the acromioclavicular joint reduced with threaded pins and to repair the coracoclavicular ligaments with fascial strips.

F. HUMERUS

1. Fracture of the Surgical Neck.

a. Manipulation usually will not appreciably improve position, especially with marked comminution (Fig. 18-2). The position is often satisfactory, although manipulation or open reduction sometimes is needed.

b. Function is the most important factor.
   1) Start early circumduction motion in a sling or collar or cuff.
   2) Hanging casts are not as comfortable, do not greatly improve alignment, and require the

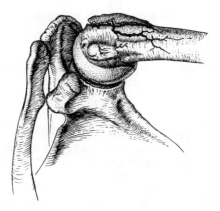

Fig. 18-2.—Humerus neck fracture.

       patient to sleep in a sitting position or with application of traction over the foot of the bed.

c. If the fracture is associated with a brachial plexus injury or dislocation of the head, *open reduction* and exploration is indicated.

2. **Shaft Fractures.**

a. In the elderly, it is often elected to apply a posterior plaster splint and sling and start early circumduction exercises to preserve function.

b. In the young patient, nonunion or malunion is fairly common. A shoulder spica should be applied to control angulation and rotation.

c. Radial nerve injury is fairly common; it may also appear later from motion at the fracture site or from *binding down* of the nerve by fracture callus.

d. Early exploration usually is *not* indicated; rely on expectant observation!

3. **Supracondylar Fracture.**

a. This fracture should be treated immediately!

b. The possibility of Volkmann's ischemic

contracture with the *five P's* warning of onset—
pain, pallor, pulselessness, paresthesia and *paralysis* of the extremity.

c. The *extension* type fracture is by far the most common.

1) The distal fragment of the humerus lies posteriorly.

2) Reduction is by longitudinal traction with the elbow in hyperextension.

3) After sufficient distraction is obtained, the distal fragment is molded forward and medial or lateral displacement or angulation is corrected.

4) The elbow is then flexed to *beyond* a right angle to maintain the reduction.

5) If the pulse disappears beyond the right angle, the patient is not a candidate for plaster immobilization and must be treated in traction.

6) If plaster immobilization is used, apply posterior plaster splints from the metacarpophalangeal joints to the axilla and use a sling.

7) If signs of impending Volkmann's contracture persist after adequate reduction, *immediately* do a stellate ganglion block.

8) If there is no improvement, *surgery is necessary at once,* not the next morning.

9) *Malunion* occurs in about 30% of the cases.

10) A change in the carrying angle of the elbow can be a cosmetic and functional disability.

11) Check the adequacy of your reduction.

a) Stand behind the patient; with his elbows flexed to 90° and at his sides, mark points at the tip of the olecranon and over both epicondyles.

b) Are the triangles on the injured and intact sides symmetrical?

c) If the apex on the injured side points *medially,* cubitus varus deformity will result.

> d) If there is an increase in *lateral* displacement of the apex, there will be increased cubitus valgus.

G. ELBOW

1. **Central Subluxation of the Head of the Radius.**
   a. This is a very common injury; the history is important.
   b. Sudden longitudinal traction has been exerted upon the upper extremity of a young child, usually under the age of three.
      1) A typical example: "I just lifted him over the curb by his hand and he started crying!"
   c. Along with his tears, the mother notes that he is not using the extremity, a form of "pseudoparalysis" due to pain.
   d. There is pain when passive flexion or extension of the elbow is attempted.
   e. The forearm is held in pronation; gentle attempts at passive supination aggravate the pain.
   f. Obtain x-ray films of the elbows, including the normal side for comparison, *before manipulation.*
   g. Quick supination of the forearm, using very little force, is all that is needed to thrust the radial head back through the annular ligament and relieve completely the painful disability. (This reduction is often accomplished by the x-ray technician in positioning the extremity for films!)
   h. Some orthopedists recommend a sling with a posterior plaster splint to hold the forearm in supination after the reduction.
      1) This is difficult to maintain in a child of this age, and is probably unnecessary.
      2) Carefully explain the mechanism of the injury to the parent!

2. **Dislocation of the Elbow.**
   a. Always check for associated neurovascular injuries.
   b. Reduce under general anesthesia.

    c. Immobilize in a posterior plaster splint with the elbow flexed beyond a right angle.

    d. If the elbow is left at a right angle, the possibility of redislocation is great.

    e. Hospitalization for several days of observation is advisable, and check films of the reduction should be obtained at 3 and 10 days.

3. Radial Head Fractures.

    a. Most will do well with immobilization until the acute pain subsides.

    b. Selected cases need surgical treatment:

        1) Marked angulation uncorrected by manipulation.

        2) Cases with marked comminution.

        3) Displaced medial marginal fractures (where osteoarthritic changes may be anticipated at the proximal radioulnar joint).

    c. These indications are for *adults*; the radial head *should never* be excised in children.

4. Olecranon Fractures.

    a. If undisplaced, the extremity may be immobilized with the elbow in 90° of flexion.

    b. Even the slightest displacement is unacceptable and open reduction with internal fixation is indicated.

5. Tennis Elbow.

    a. The patient often gives a history of repetitive exercise involving the extremity.

    b. He complains of pain localized over and distal to the lateral epicondyle of the humerus in the region of the origin of the extensor muscles.

    c. The pain may radiate down the forearm and is aggravated by pronation of the forearm, flexion of the wrist and by strong grip.

    d. Roentgenograms of the elbow are usually normal.

    e. Local injection of lidocaine with hydrocortisone (9:1) and application of a sling for several days usually relieves the pain.

f. The patient should be given analgesics for several days and *stop* playing.

g. Pain often returns after subsequent use and may require prolonged rest.

H. FOREARM

1. Radius-Ulna (Both Bone) Fractures.

a. If pronation and supination are to be preserved in the forearm, close to an anatomic reduction of both fractures is necessary.

b. In *children,* with their great growth and remodeling potential, some degree of displacement may be acceptable.

    1) Fractures of the distal 1/3 may be left in bayonet apposition and closed reduction with or without digital traction is used.

c. In *adults,* very little short of anatomic reduction can be accepted.

d. Open reduction with internal fixation is indicated if an excellent position obtained by closed reduction cannot be held in plaster.

e. This is so difficult that open reduction is the usual and accepted form of treatment for this fracture.

I. WRIST AND HAND

1. Distal Radius (Colles' Fracture).

a. There may be an assocaited ulnar styloid fracture.

b. Infiltration of the radial and ulnar fracture hematomas with lidocaine may give sufficient anesthesia for reduction.

c. General anesthesia is *much more* satisfactory for precise reduction and casting.

d. To reduce, apply longitudinal traction with countertraction to the elbow.

    1) Increase the deformity by forceable dorsiflexion of the wrist.

    2) In this position of hyperextension, the distal

       fragment can be pushed palmarward to the proper relationship with the proximal radius.

    3) The wrist is then flexed and the distal radial fragment is molded palmarward and ulnarward to correct angulation and radial displacement.

e. If the reduction is acceptable, there should be little external deformity. With both of the patient's forearms vertical, let the wrists fall into flexion. The degree of flexion should be equal.

f. Anatomic reduction by roentgenograms is not necessary for a good functional result.

g. If the reduction is lost or cannot be maintained due to comminution, healing in a displaced position causes surprisingly little disability.

h. Later, excision of the ulnar styloid is sometimes necessary for relief of pain.

i. Symptoms of median nerve compression may be present in cases with malunion.

j. A well-molded short-arm cast usually is adequate for relief of discomfort but a long-arm cast may be desirable in the comminuted fracture.

k. *It no longer* is accepted practice to place the hand in extreme palmar flexion and ulnar deviation; this may help maintain a reduction, but leaves a wrist stiff in a poor position in the older patient.

2. Navicular Fractures.

a. The patient complains of pain in the wrist, especially over the region of the anatomic snuffbox. There is pain on abduction and extension of the wrist.

b. Special, multiple angle roentgenograms may fail to demonstrate the fracture. *Any painful wrist* with *negative* roentgenograms may well be a *fracture* instead of a "sprain."

c. *Do not* treat such a case with an elastic bandage. In suspected or diagnosed navicular fractures, *apply a short arm cast* incorporating the thumb

to the interphalangeal joint in a position of abduction and opposition.

d. If initial films are negative, get check films out
of plaster at 3 weeks. Callus and resorption of
bone at the fracture site may then be very apparent. If no fracture has been sustained, your
treatment has still been *adequate and proper*
for sprain.

3. **Metacarpal Fractures (Boxer Fracture).**

a. Fractures occur at the neck of the second to
fifth metacarpals from direct trauma, as in striking a blow with the fist.

b. The most common fractures are of the fourth
and fifth metacarpals. There is palmar angulation of the metacarpal head.

c. Local infiltration of the fracture hematoma with
1% lidocaine usually provides sufficient anesthesia for reduction.

d. Flex the metacarpophalangeal and proximal interphalangeal joints to 90° and exert strong pressure over the proximal interphalangeal joint
dorsally along the axis of the proximal phalanx.

e. This may correct the angulation in a recent injury.

f. Immobilize the hand with the metacarpophalangeal and proximal interphalangeal joints of
the injured finger in 90° flexion in a short arm
cast. Do *not* immobilize the finger in *extension!*

4. **Mallet (Baseball) Finger.**

See Chapter 5, "Injuries and Infections of the Hand."

IV. THE LOWER BACK

A. LOW BACK PAIN

1. Acute low back pain has many causes. The most frequent is degenerative disc disease, with or without
herniation of disc material.

2. Evaluation may be difficult because of pain. Check

the range of motion of the spine and note any areas of splinting.
3. The neurologic examination is important. Check for:
   a. Any sensory deficit.
   b. A dermatomal pattern.
   c. Any motor deficit (long toe extensors).
   d. Test quadriceps and Achilles reflexes which should be present and symmetric.
4. Examination of the back for:
   a. Paravertebral muscle spasm.
   b. Pain upon pressure over—
      1) Spinous or transverse processes.
      2) Interspinous ligaments.
      3) Sacroiliac joints.
      4) The sciatic nerve.
   c. Record findings in the chart for later comparison.
   d. If a "trigger point" (not the sciatic nerve) is found and reproduces the same pain complained of:
      1) Infiltrate with 10 ml. of lidocaine, 1%.
      2) If complete relief is obtained, the test has been therapeutic and diagnostic.
      3) Probably rules out a herniated disc.
   e. If a diagnosis of herniated disc is suspected, or if the diagnosis is not clear, the patient may be given analgesics and put on bedrest with bathroom privileges at home.
   f. It may be necessary to admit the patient to the hospital for complete bedrest, relief of pain and additional tests.

V. THE HIP

A. FRACTURES

1. These may occur with little or no trauma in the elderly.
2. The shortened lower extremity lies in external rotation (greater in intertrochanteric than in neck fractures).

3. Movement at the hip causes groin or knee pain.
4. There is pain on pressure over the greater trochanter.
5. The intertrochanteric type may result in several units of blood extravasating into the thigh, an increase in thigh circumference and shock.
6. Most neck and intertrochanteric fractures are best treated by reduction and internal fixation.
7. The primary use of prosthesis may be best in the elderly patient with a neck fracture.
8. Comminuted intertrochanteric fractures may not have sufficient stability for internal fixation. Traction, therefore, will be required.
9. Surgery is usually the conservative treatment in hip fractures.
    a. The patient is out of bed soon after surgery.
    b. Has fewer pulmonary complications.
    c. Has a lower morbidity and mortality rate.
    d. The patient gets home sooner.
    e. Buck's adhesive traction is often used until the patient is ready for surgery.

B. HIP DISLOCATIONS

1. Sciatic nerve injury is sometimes associated.
2. Early reduction is imperative and lessens such complications as late aseptic necrosis of the femoral head or pressure injury of the sciatic nerve.

C. TROCHANTERIC BURSITIS

1. The main problem is confusion with true hip disease or with herniated intervertebral disc in those cases having radiation of pain into the lower extremity from the bursitis.
2. Either the subcutaneous or, more commonly, the deep trochanteric bursa may be involved.
3. Direct pressure over the bursa duplicates the pain, which is usually an aseptic bursitis.
4. If there are no signs of infection, 5 ml. of 1% lidocaine with 10 mg. of hydrocortisone can be injected into the bursa.

5. This usually will confirm the diagnosis by relief of pain and is therapeutic.

VI. THE LOWER EXTREMITY

A. FEMORAL SHAFT

1. Diaphyseal Fractures.

a. As in intertrochanteric fractures, there may be appreciable blood loss into the thigh.
b. Fat embolism may occur.
c. Eyegrounds and urine must be examined.
d. An associated vascular or neurologic injury indicates internal fixation.
e. This fracture can be managed adequately by careful traction.
f. Open reduction and internal fixation gets the patient up and around sooner.
g. The rate of healing is not increased.
h. The risk of infection and nonunion as well as the morbidity and mortality of any surgical procedure and general anesthesia must be considered.

2. Supracondylar Fractures.

a. Popliteal artery injury may be a complication.
b. The best functional result usually is obtained by meticulous traction with a tibial pin and balanced suspension (see Chap. 12 and p. 286).

B. THE KNEE

1. Patellar Fractures.

a. Undisplaced "crack" fractures may be immobilized with the knee in extension.
b. Check films are taken at 3 and 10 days.
c. If the fragments are separated, surgical reduction is required.

2. Internal Derangements.

a. A thorough history is extremely important.
b. A common injury is a torn medial meniscus,

sometimes associated with anterior cruciate and medial collateral ligament tears.

   1) A typical history is of sudden onset of pain following internal rotation of the femur upon the fixed tibia and foot (as in football).

c. If swelling was slow, over a period of hours, a serous effusion is likely; anticipate a cartilage injury only.

d. If the swelling was rapid, anticipate ligament tears or a fracture with a hemarthrosis.

e. Young girls may dislocate the patella laterally.

f. This may spontaneously reduce leaving only slight swelling and pain on pressure around the medial margin of the patella.

g. The patient will resist lateral motion of the patella with the knee flexed (motion may be abnormally increased).

h. Any acute knee injury may cause sufficient pain to prevent thorough examination. The patient may require examination under anesthesia.

   1) Under strict aseptic conditions, aspirate the knee and inject 5 ml. of lidocaine through the same needle.

   2) Note if the aspirated fluid is serous or bloody. Let the tube of fluid stand.

   3) If globules of fat (marrow) rise to the surface, anticipate an osteochondral fracture which may *not* be apparent on roentgenograms!

   4) With the knee flexed at $15°$, check for abnormal *mobility* with medial or lateral pressure applied to the lower leg. If a medial or lateral collateral ligament is torn, excessive motion will be felt and a fingertip on the joint line will feel the joint rock open on the injured side.

   5) Test for excess *anteroposterior* motion of the head of the tibia with the knee flexed to $90°$. Excessive anterior motion of the tibia is possible with a torn anterior cruciate

ligament and excessive posterior motion with the much less common tear of the posterior cruciate ligament.

    i. Many tests are described to demonstrate torn cartilages, but none is exceptionally reliable. The leg may be held in full internal or external rotation with the knee acutely flexed.

        1) A snap or click is sometimes felt or heard as the knee is then brought into full extension while maintaining the rotation of the leg. There are many variations and eponyms for such tests.

        2) Abnormal laxity, "pops," "clicks" or other findings may be bilateral and unrelated to the injury.

    j. Attempt to establish a diagnosis promptly. Diagnosis will be more difficult later after immobilization in a cylinder or after use of crutches.

    k. Obtain adequate roentgenograms of the knee; these should include "tunnel" or intercondylar notch views and "skyline" or tangential views of the patella in addition to the usual lateral and anteroposterior views.

    l. A diagnosis of a torn meniscus or a loose body usually warrants early surgery.

    m. Intensive quadriceps drills, graduating from isometric to progressive resistance, is the key to recovery after any knee surgery.

    n. Early surgical repair usually is advised for torn collateral ligaments. Repair of cruciate ligament tears is of questionable value.

3. **Tibial Plateau Fractures.**

    a. Some fractures with a single large fragment warrant open reduction with internal fixation after the plateau is elevated.

    b. Most will do quite well after closed reduction of the fracture followed by early range of motion exercises in balanced suspension.

    c. The functional result often will be better than

one might expect on evaluation of roentgeno-grams alone.

4. **Chondromalacia of the Patella.**
   a. The patient may be able to give a history of re-cent or old trauma to the patella, but the disease can occur due to continued normal use.
   b. The pathologic process is a degenerative change of the articular surface of the patella, which is really only a part of a more generalized change in the entire knee.
   c. The patient complains of pain fairly well local-ized to the anterior aspect of the knee. The pain is aggravated by climbing and descending the stairs and often does not appear until late in the day.
      1) With the patient relaxed and supine, and the knee extended, crepitus may be felt as the patella is passively glided over the femoral condyles.
      2) Pain will most certainly be felt if the patella is pulled distally, pressure applied in a pos-terior direction on the patella and the pa-tient then asked to contract the quadriceps.
   d. This is not an emergency situation, but it must be distinguished from other acute injuries to the knee.

C. TIBIAL SHAFT FRACTURE

1. Most can be treated satisfactorily by closed reduc-tion.
   a. Associated vascular injury probably occurs more often than is suspected clinically; collaterals us-ually suffice. *Vascular* injury takes *priority* in treatment.
2. These fractures should be reduced under general anesthesia if the position is not satisfactory.
3. With the knee flexed to 90° over the edge of the table, traction on the foot and ankle with direct pressure applied over the fracture usually will

afford acceptable alignment and rotation.

4. With the knee still flexed, apply a well-molded short leg cast. When this has hardened, it can be extended to a long leg cast with the knee in about 10° of flexion without losing position.

5. The prognosis should be discussed with the patient. Proximal shaft fractures are through cancellous bone and usually heal with no difficulty. Fractures through the *distal third* are in an area of poor blood supply; delayed union is common and nonunion is by no means rare. Prolonged immobilization may be necessary in this case, sometimes for 6-9 months.

D. THE ANKLE

1. **Sprain.**

   a. The anterior talofibular ligament is the most commonly injured and there will be point tenderness anterior to the lateral malleolus.

   b. Do *not* make the diagnosis without roentgenograms of the ankle! Films should include:
      1) An internal rotation (oblique or mortise) view to demonstrate congruity of talus and articular surfaces of the tibia and fibula.
      2) An additional oblique view with the foot held in an inverted position with some stress applied. The injection of local anesthetic may be necessary.

   c. If this view (Fig. 18-3) shows the talus to be significantly tilted in mortise, open repair of the ligamentous injury usually is advisable.

   d. For the uncomplicated sprain, elastic bandages and taping are sometimes used in treatment, but the patient ambulates with discomfort and pain. Crutches with nonweight bearing are comfortable, but have obvious disadvantages.

   e. Immediate application of a short leg walking cast will allow the patient full, painless weight bearing and minimal fatigue from the altered gait.

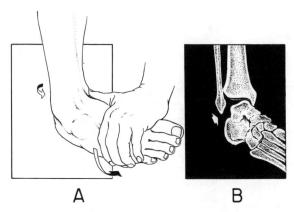

Fig. 18-3.—Ankle injury. Oblique view with foot held in inverted position.

    f.   The cast is removed in 2-3 weeks and followed with an Unna boot for a week or so to prevent swelling as activity is resumed. The patient can remove the boot himself.

    g.   Local heat is never indicated in the acute stage of the injury. It will only increase the swelling.

2. **Fractures.**

    a.   The history of the mechanism of injury is very helpful. If the mechanism of injury is reversed, adequate reduction is often obtained even after gross displacement.

    b.   Films must include A.P., lateral and mortise (oblique) views. The "clear space" around the talus should be of the same width on both sides and top.

    c.   Early reduction before swelling and bleb formation occur is important. Some cases will require open reduction.

    d.   Check films should be taken at 3 and 10 days to be certain that reduction has been maintained.

Prolonged disability and secondary traumatic arthritis are the sequelae of failure.

E. THE FOOT

1. Os Calcis Fractures.

a. Check for associated compression fractures of the spine if the mechanism of injury was a fall from a height.

b. Opinion is divided as to whether either open *or* closed reduction is indicated. It is sometimes elected to mold gross crush with heel varus or valgus into a better position under general anesthesia.

c. The best results seem to follow elevation of the extremity after application of pressure dressings. When the swelling and most of the acute pain have subsided, early weight bearing (with or without a short leg walking cast) will further mold the fracture fragments into the best possible position for function. Here, as in most fractures, function is the foremost consideration. Don't treat a roentgenogram!

2. Fracture of Base of the Fifth Metatarsal.

a. The peroneus brevis muscle inserts on the base of the fifth metatarsal. The mechanism of injury is the avulsion of the base of the metatarsal by a sharp, sudden contraction of the muscle as sometimes happens during a misstep.

b. It is a common injury often confused with a sprained ankle. The tenderness and swelling is around the fifth metatarsal base, not around the anterior tip of the lateral maleolus!

c. These patients are often reasonably comfortable in ordinary street shoes. If pain during walking is great, the patient may need a short leg walking cast.

3. Phalangeal Fractures.

a. Firm, well-fitting shoes relieve much of the pain during walking.

    b. Taping adjacent toes together helps *little* with relief of pain and may lead to problems of skin maceration unless adequate padding is placed between the toes.

VII. TRACTION

A. **BUCK'S EXTENSION.**—This is skin traction with moleskin tape.

    1. It can be applied to any extremity, but is probably most frequently used for temporary immobilization after hip fractures.

    2. Tincture of benzoin is applied from the toes to the knee. The extremity is not shaved as this often leads to folliculitis and lessens the adherence of the tape.

    3. Several layers of sheet wadding are applied from the toes to just above the malleoli to protect these bone prominences. Moleskin tapes are applied from below the knee to the upper margin of the sheet wadding. These specially made tapes have webbing-belts attached to their lower ends.

    4. The belts are then temporarily turned back up toward the knee and an elastic bandage is loosely applied circumferentially over the sheet wadding from the toes to the lower margin of the tapes (Fig. 18-4).

    5. The belts are then again turned distally and the elastic bandage continued over the tapes up to the knee, no stretch is applied. The end of the bandage is secured with several pieces of tape and the webbing-belts are threaded through the medial and lateral buckles of the foot plate and secured. The traction eye on the underside of the foot plate is located just anterior to the axis of the ankle joint.

    6. When 5-10 pounds of weight is applied through rope over a pulley at the foot of the bed, traction is applied and the foot is simultaneously held in dorsiflexion to prevent equinus contracture. The foot of

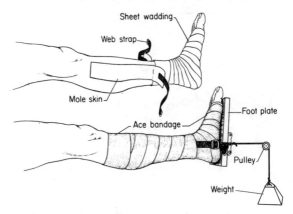

Fig. 18-4.—Buck's extension.

the bed may be elevated 6 inches if the patient tends to shift down in the bed.

7. Other typical applications of moleskin traction are used in balanced suspension (also to prevent equinus) and in Dunlop's traction for supracondylar fractures of the humerus.

B. BALANCED SUSPENSION WITH THOMAS SPLINT AND PEARSON ATTACHMENT

1. Balanced suspension can be used to partially immobilize a lower extremity while maintaining mobility of the joints.

2. A Thomas splint is used. If it is a half-ring, the ring should lie across the groin, rather than posteriorly in the gluteal fold where it may cause discomfort. A narrow strip of tape laid longitudinally on the outside rod of the splint will provide a surface on which the toweling used will not slip.

3. The splint is set in place with its axis at the level of the knee joint (Fig. 18-5).

4. Folded towels are then passed around the medial

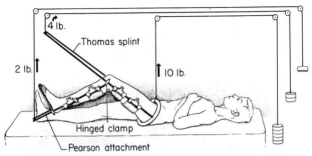

Fig. 18-5.—Balanced suspension with Thomas splint and Pearson attachment.

rod of the splint and under the thigh thence over the lateral rod where they are clipped in place. The same routine is followed below the knee, but now on the rods of the Pearson attachment.

5. The patient will be more comfortable if a 3-inch strip of felt, covered with stocking, is placed on the toweling to run from the gluteal fold to the upper edge of the heelcord. This prevents wrinkled toweling from touching the skin.

6. In a typical case for an adult, the splint can then be suspended from an overhead frame with 4 pounds of weight for the distal end of the Thomas splint, 10 pounds for the proximal end and 2 pounds for the end of the Pearson attachment. The ropes are led to overhead pulleys and thence to pulleys either at the head (preferred) or foot of the bed where the weights are suspended.

7. A typical application for this suspension would be after reduction of a trumatic dislocation of the hip. It is often used after hip surgery. It can be combined with skeletal traction or, for femoral shaft fractures, with distal femoral or proximal tibial pins. It may be useful, with modifications, in other fractures.

CHAPTER 19

Pediatric Medical Emergencies

JO ANN M. CORNET, M.D.

I. EVALUATION OF THE FEBRILE CHILD

Children are brought to the Emergency Service for a variety of signs and symptoms. While most Emergency Service visits are not in the true sense medical or surgical emergencies, it should be recognized that serious illnesses in the child, and especially the young infant, are often characterized by an extremely abrupt onset which may have as the *only sign* the presence of *fever*.

Important accompanying symptoms may be refusal to feed, vomiting, diarrhea, unusual fussiness or lethargy. Fever of unknown origin (FUO) is one of the most frequently encountered problems in an emergency.

Failure to elicit a complete history, perform a thorough physical examination and order appropriate laboratory tests may result in unnecessary morbidity and/or mortality.

The discharge of an infant or a young child with the diagnosis of "FUO-probably an incipient viral illness" is *not justifiable* unless adequate investigation of *each child* has been conducted satisfactorily. If physical examination fails to reveal a focus of infection, the following approach is suggested.

A. INFANTS IN THE NEWBORN PERIOD

1. Sepsis, meningitis or urinary tract infection should be strongly suspected, and such infants should be admitted to the hospital.
2. Appropriate diagnostic studies (including lumbar puncture, blood culture, chest x-ray film, urinalysis and CBC) should be initiated and therapy instituted promptly.

3. *Specific* clinical signs and symptoms are often *absent* in the infant under 3 months of age.

B. OLDER INFANTS AND CHILDREN UNDER AGE 3 YEARS

1. Inability of the patient to communicate symptomatology, e.g., headache, earache, sore throat, abdominal pain, is characteristic of this age group.
2. If the physical examination is negative, investigation should include:
   a. Chest x-ray film, since auscultatory findings may be unimpressive even in the presence of bronchopneumonia.
   b. Microscopic examination of a clean voided urine sample.
   c. Microscopic examination, methylene blue and gram stain of cerebral spinal fluid.
   d. If the lumbar puncture is traumatic, the fluid still should be cultured.
3. It is *strongly recommended* that the infant be admitted to the hospital for observation and/or a repeat spinal tap. Although the white blood count and differential can be misleading in determining whether a fever is of bacterial or viral origin, the CBC may often aid in selecting further diagnostic studies.
4. Alcohol sponging is indicated for temperature over 103°F. and aspirin (65 mg. per year of age) as symptomatic treatment while the child is being evaluated.

C. OLDER CHILDREN

The older child with fever often is able to relate a specific complaint. While meticulous attention to the details of the history and physical examination is essential, diagnostic laboratory studies are less important in the older child. However, a urinalysis and a tuberculin test may reveal the source of FUO.

II. MANAGEMENT OF SPECIFIC SYMPTOMS
IN CHILDREN

A. DEHYDRATION

1. Dehydration, often with accompanying *electrolyte imbalance,* may result from a variety of causes in previously well children (decreased fluid intake, increased gastrointestinal loss from vomiting or diarrhea).
2. It may also occur in children with predisposing diseases:
   a. Cystic fibrosis.
   b. Adrenocortical insufficiency.
   c. Diabetes mellitus.
   d. Diabetes insipidus.
3. Unless there is good evidence of excessive fluid intake or a high solute load that leads one to suspect either hypotonic or hypertonic dehydration, it is reasonable to assume *initially* that *isotonic* dehydration exists.
4. Obtain accurate weight with patient undressed.
5. Start I.V. fluids in most accessible vein, and obtain blood sample for electrolytes (Na, K. Cl, CO_2, pH) and other chemistries which appear to be indicated (glucose, serum acetone, BUN, salicylate level).
6. *Administer* half-strength saline in 5% glucose and water, 20 ml./kg., rapidly (30-60 minutes).
7. If the patient appears to be more than 10% dehydrated, has a rapid pulse, and is hyperventilating, 1/6 M.Na. lactate, 20 ml./kg. should be given as the *initial* hydrating fluid.
8. If the patient is in SHOCK, give plasma, 10 ml./kg., as rapidly as possible to restore circulation.
9. Critical time may be lost in an effort to perform a venipuncture in a young child in shock. Obtain blood chemistries *after* patient is out of shock.
10. If several attempts are not successful, fluids may be infused through a no. 18 needle directly into the bone marrow of the tibia (in an infant under 1 year

of age), or in the iliac crest, intraperitoneally, or via a saphenous vein cutdown.

11. After the circulation has improved, blood may be obtained for chemical analysis and conventional sites for administration of fluids usually can be utilized.

12. While awaiting the results of the blood chemistries, follow the initial fluids with a *1:2:3 solution* (*1* part 1/6 M.Na. lactate, *2* parts normal saline, *3* parts 5% glucose and water) at the rate of 10 ml./kg./hour.

13. Place a urine collection device on the patient as soon as possible while fluids are being given.

B. CONVULSIONS

1. Convulsions at the onset or during a febrile illness occur frequently in young (less than 2-3 years of age) children and may or may not indicate a central nervous system infection.

2. A convulsion in an afebrile child can be due to a *variety of causes:*
   a. Metabolic disorders.
      1) Electrolyte imbalance.
      2) Hypoglycemia.
      3) Hypocalcemia.
   b. Intoxication.
      1) Lead.
      2) Phenothiazine.
   c. Intracranial hemorrhage.
      1) Vascular accidents.
      2) Coagulation disturbances.
   d. Brain tumor.
   e. Cerebral defects.
   f. Degenerative diseases.
   g. Hypertensive encephalopathy (acute glomerulonephritis).
   h. Idiopathic epilepsy.

3. *Immediate management* of the child during the convulsion consists of:
   a. Protection with a mouth gag, suctioning secretions, padding and restraining when necessary.

      b. Giving *Diazepam* (Valium) 2-10 mg., I.V. slowly until seizure stops.

      c. Alcohol sponging for elevated temperature.

4. As soon as the seizure is controlled, or if the child is first seen in a postictal condition, a thorough history and physical examination are performed to attempt to determine the etiology of the convulsion.

5. In addition to a lumbar puncture, it is advisable to *admit* any child with his first convulsion to the hospital for diagnostic studies.

6. Febrile children with a history of previous febrile convulsions should be assessed carefully and lumbar puncture performed unless the cause of the fever is apparent.

C. CROUP (LARYNGEAL STRIDOR)

1. Croup in infants and children usually is due to a viral upper respiratory infection.

2. Acute epiglottiditis and laryngotracheobronchitis may be caused by H. influenza.

3. In the absence of infection, stridor may occur from laryngeal edema secondary to trauma, allergy or from laryngeal obstruction from a *foreign body*.

4. Certain children have a tendency to develop recurrent stridor in association with respiratory infection. In these children, fever usually is not markedly elevated ($100°$-$102°$), and high humidity administered at home usually controls the symptoms.

5. The child having his initial episode of croup who appears ill, is markedly febrile ($> 103°$) and has had symptoms which increase or persist despite efforts at home, *should be hospitalized* for both supportive and antimicrobial therapy.

6. Tracheostomy may be indicated (see Chap. 23, "Otolaryngologic Emergencies").

7. Changes in pulse rate and respirations should be observed carefully; the child who appears to be tiring and has decreasing respiratory exchange should be evaluated for tracheostomy *before* cyanosis appears.

D. ASTHMA

Mild to moderately severe wheezing frequently can be controlled with:
1. Aqueous epinephrine (1:1000) 0.01 ml./kg. per dose, s.c. (maximum single dose not to exceed 0.5 ml.). However, this is contraindicated in a "dry" asthmatic.
2. If 2 doses of epinephrine do not terminate the attack, aminophylline 3.5 mg./kg. diluted with 150-200 cc. 5% D/W should be administered *slowly*, I.V.
3. Concomitant administration of I.V. fluids to liquefy mucus is beneficial, and is especially important if the child is dehydrated.
4. If the above measures do not abate attack, the patient should be admitted to the hospital.

E. BRONCHIOLITIS

Bronchiolitis, a frequent manifestation of respiratory infection in infants under age 2 years, is characterized by:
1. The rapid development of generalized obstructive emphysema.
2. Prolongation of expiration with wheezing and occasionally rales.
3. *Small infants* can develop severe respiratory distress with poor ventilatory exchange *rapidly*.
4. Specific supportive measures to ensure high humidity and adequate hydration are necessary, and *hospitalization* is recommended.

F. ACUTE ADRENOCORTICAL INSUFFICIENCY

1. Acute adrenocortical insufficiency may occur in a child with chronic adrenal insufficiency who undergoes stress from a superimposed acute illness with:
   a. Fever.
   b. Vomiting.
   c. Diarrhea.
2. Profound disturbances of fluid and electrolyte balance may result.
3. **Treatment.**
   a. Solu-Cortef: 60-150 mg. I.V.

b. I.V. fluids: 5% dextrose in normal saline.
c. DOCA: 2-4 mg. I.M. (unless, by history, DOCA has been given in previous 24 hours).
d. Determination of serum electrolytes with subsequent specific replacement.

G. CARDIOPULMONARY ARREST (see Chap. 1)

1. Although the absence of respiration usually is obvious, the absence of functional circulation may not be.
2. The heart may be beating feebly with such minimal cardiac output that oxygenation of vital centers is inadequate.
3. *Immediate therapy* consists of re-establishing adequate ventilation and circulation.
4. Establish ventilation immediately.
   a. Open airway by cleaning out mouth, and hyperextend neck.
   b. Apply mouth-to-mouth or mouth-to-airway expired air ventilation. This is done by pinching the nostrils of the patient and exhaling into mouth or airway so that chest is seen to expand.
   c. Resuscitator then withdraws mouth, takes another breath, allowing air to leave patient.
   d. This procedure is repeated every *4-5 seconds* (12-15 times per minute).
5. Immediately establish artificial circulation with external (manual) heart compression.
   a. With the patient on a firm surface, place thumbs (with small infant) or heel of hand (with an older child) on the lower end of the sternum and apply firm pressure, depressing sternum 1-2 inches for about 1/2 second, releasing and reapplying at the rate of 80-100 times per minute.
6. Immediately summon assistance.
7. Necessary equipment—ECG, defibrillator and cardiotonic drugs—should be immediately available in every emergency service ("crash" cart). Establish if circulatory arrest is due to ventricular standstill or fibrillation. Continue assisting ventilation and circulation.

8. **Standstill** (see Chap. 1).
   a. Slap precordium.
   b. Cardiac puncture.
   c. External cardiac pacemaker.
   d. Administration of cardiotonic or vasopressor drugs.
      1) Epinephrine, I.V.: 1 *mg.* in 250 ml. normal saline.
      2) Epinephrine, intracardiac: 2-3 *ml.* of 1:10,000 dilution.
      3) Calcium chloride, intracardiac: 3-5 ml. of a 10% solution.
      4) Sodium bicarbonate (50 mEq./50 ml.): 2 mEq/kg. I.V. for metabolic acidosis; repeat in 15-20 minutes as necessary.
9. **Fibrillation**: Apply electric countershock with cardiac defibrillator.
10. **Cardiac failure** (congestive heart failure).
    a. Obtain accurate weight, with patient undressed.
    b. Administer oxygen.
    c. Digitalize with digoxin: *Total digitalizing dose.*
       1) Infants under 10 kg.: 0.08 mg./kg.
       2) Children 10-25 kg.: 0.06 mg./kg.
       3) Children over 25 kg.: 0.04 mg./kg.
       4) Give one-half total dose stat I.M.
       5) Give one-fourth total dose in next 6-8 hours; remaining one-fourth dose 6-8 hours later.
       6) *Maintenance dose: one-fourth* total digitalizing dose.
    d. Obtain ECG prior to and during digitalization.
    e. Diuretic: *Thiomerin (I.M.)* in following dosages:
       1) Infants 6-15 *lb.*: 0.12-0.25 ml.
       2) Children 15-30 *lb.*: 0.25-0.50 ml.
       3) Older children: 0.50-1.5 ml.

III. DIABETES

A. HYPOGLYCEMIC COMA

1. Draw blood for glucose and electrolyte levels.

2. Administer glucagon, 0.1 mg./kg., not to exceed 1.0 mg.
3. Administer a 50% glucose solution (1-2 cc./kg.) I.V., followed by 10% glucose.

B. DIABETIC COMA

1. Draw blood for glucose, CO_2, Na, Cl, K, BUN, pH and serum acetone levels. (Use Acetest tablets, also).
2. Administer crystalline insulin, 2.0 units/kg. *Give one-half dose I.V., one-half dose s.c.*
3. Begin I.V. fluids:
   a. 20 cc./kg. of 1/6 M.Na. lactate over a 1-2-hour period.
   b. Follow with a *1:2:3 solution* (1 part 1/6 M.Na. lactate, 2 parts normal saline, 3 parts 5% D/W).
4. Wash out stomach with one-half normal saline if abdomen is distended.
5. Follow serum acetone (Acetest tablet) and blood glucose (Dextrostix) every 2 hours.
6. Repeat insulin: 0.5-1.0 unit/kg. in 4-6 hours.
7. Repeat chemistries in 4-6 hours.
8. Analyze each urine sample for reducing sugar and acetone. (Do not forget to do complete urinalysis on *initial specimen*.)

IV. MANAGEMENT OF SPECIFIC INFECTIOUS DISEASES

A. MENINGOCOCCEMIA

1. The clinical impression of acute meningococcemia constitutes an urgent situation in which prompt institution of proper therapy is critical.
2. Draw blood for culture, CBC, and coagulation studies.
3. Follow *immediately* with aqueous penicillin, 1,000,000 units I.V., and every 2 hours thereafter.
4. Since it has been demonstrated that fulminant meningococcemia can be complicated by *intravascular*

coagulation, all such patients should be evaluated for this possibility. Screening tests that may indicate the presence of intravascular clotting are:

a. Low platelet count or diminished platelets on peripheral smear.

b. Prolonged prothrombin time.

c. Prolonged partial thromboplastin time.

d. Low fibrinogen on screening test (Fi test).

e. Specific coagulation factor assays (factor V, factor VIII and fibrinogen) may give further support to the abnormal findings from screening tests.

f. Although the role of heparin has not been definitely established, it has been suggested that heparinization may be beneficial in the presence of intravascular clotting in meningococcemia.

g. If used, heparin should be given I.V., 100 units/kg. every 4 hours until coagulation has returned to normal.

5. If the patient is in SHOCK, or if vital signs indicate impending shock, circulation should be supported with plasma or whole blood, 10-20 ml./kg.

6. Hydrocortisone, 50-100 mg./kg. I.V. may also be useful in treating *endotoxic* shock. Repeat every 6 hours.

B. MENINGITIS

1. Acute purulent meningitis requires prompt management not only to decrease mortality, but to diminish subsequent morbidity.

2. The gram stain is usually negative because inadequate antibiotic treatment already has been started.

3. *Until* the results of cerebospinal fluid and blood *cultures* are available, immediate therapy consists of:

a. In the *infant* under 3 months of age: ampicillin 50 mg./kg., *stat* and *I.V.* every 8 hours and kanamycin, 15 mg./kg. *stat* and 7.5 mg./kg. *I.M.* every 12 hours.

b. After age 3 months: ampicillin, 50 mg./kg. I.V. every 6 hours.

    c. After bacteriologic identification, the following agents are substituted:
  1) *Meningococcus:* Aqueous crystalline penicillin, 1,000,000 units I.V. every 2 hours.
  2) *Pneumococcus:* Aqueous crystalline penicillin, 1,000,000 units I.V. every 2 hours.
  3) *H. influenzae:* Continue ampicillin, 50 mg./kg. I.V. every 6 hours.
  4) *Staphylococcus:* Methicillin, 100 mg./kg. I.V. every 6 hours.
  5) *Streptococcus:* Aqueous crystalline penicillin, 1,000,000 units I.V. every 2 hours.

C. PNEUMONIA

1. Undress the infant or young child and observe his respirations.
2. Subtle physical signs of flaring of nasal alae, costal retractions and tachypnea are often obscured by crying.
3. Slightly diminished *breath-sounds* may be the only finding.
4. The physician's *index of suspicion* should be high, and a prompt roentgenographic examination of the chest is indicated.
5. If signs and symptoms of pneumonia are present, hospitalization is indicated for:
   a. Infants less than 1 year of age.
   b. Any infant or child with moderate to severe respiratory distress and/or evidence of pleural effusion.
   c. Any child under age 3 with a *previous* history of pneumonia.
   d. Any child with a predisposing illness such as:
      1) Sickle cell anemia.
      2) Fibrocystic disease.
      3) Diabetes mellitus.
      4) Agammaglobulinemia.
6. **Treatment.**—Procaine penicillin 600,000 units I.M. daily for 5 days is the treatment of choice.

7. Children with pneumonia *should be followed close-ly.*
8. Other causes must be considered depending upon:
    a. Roentgenographic findings.
    b. Smear and culture of sputum.
    c. The clinical course.
9. A tuberculin skin test is indicated.

D. TONSILLITIS AND PHARYNGITIS

Tonsillitis and pharyngitis are among the most fre-quently encountered pediatric illnesses. An accurate diagnosis (viral vs. streptococcal) cannot be made on the basis of the clinical impression alone.

1. Obtain a throat culture.
2. Treat symptomatically with ASA until the culture is reported.
3. If beta Hemolytic Streptococcus (Group A) is found, *treat with:*
    a. Benzathine penicillin (Bicillin) 600,000 units I.M. (single dose) or
    b. Penicillin 600,000 units I.M. daily, then orally for 10 days.
    c. In patients *allergic* to penicillin, erythromycin 40-50 mg./kg. in 4 divided doses daily for 10 days is the drug of choice (see "Antibiotics," Part I, 4).

E. OTITIS MEDIA (see "Antibiotics," Part I, 4)

1. Otitis media is a common childhood infection.
2. Differentiation between acute purulent otitis media and serous otitis media is often difficult.
3. If any doubt exists, it is advisable to initiate anti-microbial therapy in addition to nasal decongestants.
4. Since the majority of cases of purulent otitis media are due to penicillin-sensitive organisms (pneumo-coccus, streptococcus) and since a large percentage of H. influenzae organisms are also penicillin sensi-tive, PENICILLIN is the drug of choice. *Dosage:* 600,000 units I.M., *stat,* followed by 400,000 units, orally for 10 days.

F. IMPETIGO

1. Impetigo is a frequent dermatologic problem seen in the Emergency Service. The rapidity of the spread of these lesions is alarming to the parents.
2. *Culture* usually reveals a mixture of staphylococcus and streptococcus.
3. Since the poststreptococcal sequel of acute glomerulonephritis has occurred following impetigo, it is advisable to prescribe both local and systemic therapy.
4. *Obtain culture* after removing part of the crust from the lesion.
5. Instruct parents in *local* hygiene: Phisohex scrubs to infected areas, manicure, and scrub nail beds.
6. Administration of benzathine penicillin, 600,000 units, usually will eradicate both organisms.
7. Topical ointments (e.g., bacitracin) provide a local bactericidal effect.

G. MANAGEMENT OF PEDIATRIC ALLERGIC MANIFESTATIONS (see "Allergic Emergencies," Chap. 25).

Allergic reactions in children can present a wide spectrum of clinical manifestations ranging from mild urticaria, generalized angioneurotic edema to anaphylaxis.

1. Urticaria (hives) are usually relieved by:
    a. Benadryl 1.0-1.5 mg./kg. either P.O. or I.V. every hour. If response is incomplete,
    b. Aqueous epinephrine 1:1000, 0.01 ml./kg., s.c. (maximum dose 0.5 cc.). The above dose may be repeated in 4 hours.
    c. Corticosteroids generally tend to act more slowly than the above agents; steroid therapy can be used in addition to the other agents in severe or prolonged urticaria. In these cases, *hospitalization* is indicated.
2. Angioneurotic edema.
    a. Angioneurotic edema can be especially threatening in a young child in whom the airway easily can be compromised.

    b.   Treatment consists of the *same* agents as in urticaria (see above). However, the *route of administration should be I.V.*

3. Anaphylaxis.
    a.   The precipitous onset makes extremely rapid action mandatory.
    b.   If anaphylaxis develops consequent to a therapeutic agent, or to an insect sting (Hymenoptera are the most frequent offenders), a tourniquet proximal to the site may delay further systemic absorption.
    c.   Epinephrine, 1:1000, 0.25 cc. directly into the site of entry may also produce local delay of absorption of the offending agent.
    d.   In addition to measures suggested for angioneurotic edema, *cardiopulmonary resuscitation,* (Chap. 1) may be required.

V. PHYSICAL ABUSE OF CHILDREN (THE BATTERED CHILD)

A. During the past several years, there has been growing appreciation of the problem of the physically abused child (the so-called "battered child"). These children commonly are identified by the finding of multiple bone injuries on x-ray film in the *absence* of specific bone disease, a history of trauma or the presence of multiple ecchymoses in the *absence* of a blood dyscrasia. There often is evidence of neglect.

B. It is recognized that the parents of such children have severe emotional problems which require professional help and that the children require protection while the family situation is assessed. The mortality rate and incidence of permanent physical and mental damage is *high* in physically abused children.

C. *Children who are suspected of being physically abused should be hospitalized immediately and the case referred to Social Service for study. The Police should <u>not</u> be notified.*

D. *The parent or guardian should not be questioned about or accused of physical abuse,* since this usually is denied and may result in removal of the child from medical care.

E. Many such children will be seen first by a surgeon in the Emergency Service; the parents often volunteer a history of accidental injury. However, a pediatrician should be contacted immediately if there is any suspicion of physical abuse. Admission to the hospital should be arranged and the appropriate social service and legal agencies contacted.

VI. THE PEDIATRIC DOSAGE OF DRUGS

A. The doses given below usually are based on *body weight in kilograms (1 kg. = 2.2 lb.)*

1. *Apresoline:*	0.15 ml./kg. given as a single dose *with Reserpine,* .07 mg./kg. every 12-24 hours for *hypertension.*
2. *Aminophylline:*	Intravenously: 12-15 mg./kg. per 24 hours. Divide into 4-6 doses. Rectally: Double the above dose.
3. *Aspirin:*	65 mg. (1 grain) per year of age every 6 hours *or* 65 mg./kg. per 24 hours *not to exceed* 325 mg. or 5 grains per dose.
4. *Benadryl:*	5 mg./kg. per 24 hours. Divide into 4 doses.
5. *Chloral hydrate:*	50 mg./kg. per 24 hours. Do not exceed 1 Gm. in single dose.
6. *Codeine:*	For pain: 3 mg./kg. per 24 hours. Divide into 6 doses. *Cough syrups* can contain *8-10* mg. per teaspoonful (5 ml.)
7. *Compazine:*	0.4 mg./kg. per 24 hours. Divide into 4 doses.
8. *Demerol:*	6.0 mg./kg. per 24 hours. Divide into 6 doses.

9. *Diazepam (Valium):* 2-10 mg. I.V., slowly until convulsion stops.

10. *Digoxin:* *Digitalizing dose*
    a. Infants under 10 kg.: 0.08 mg./kg.
    b. Children 10-25 kg.: 0.06 mg./kg.
    c. Children over 25 kg.: 0.04 mg./kg.
    d. Give *one-half* total dose *I.M. stat*; give one-fourth total dose in next 6-8 hours; give remaining one-fourth dose 6-8 hours later.
    e. *Maintenance*—one-fourth of total digitalizing dose.

11. *Dilantin:* 4-6 mg./kg. per 24 hours. Divide into 2-3 doses.

12. *Dramamine:* 5 mg./kg. per 24 hours. Divide into 4 doses.

13. *Ephedrine sulfate:* 3 mg./kg. per 24 hours. Divide into 4-6 doses.

14. *Epinephrine:*
    a. 0.01 ml./kg. per dose of 1:1000 solution. Maximum single dose 0.05 ml.
    b. Repeat every 4 hours parenterally. For I.V. infusion, 1:10,000 is used.

15. *Gamma globulin:*
    a. Measles, preventive dose: 0.22 ml./kg.
    b. Measles, attenuating dose: 0.05 ml./kg.
    c. Hepatitis, preventive dose: 0.02 mg./kg.

16. *Ipecac syrup:* 15 ml. orally. May be repeated once in 30 minutes if emesis has not occurred. *Note:* Use syrup *only*.

17. *Levophed:*   1.0 ml. of 0.2% solution diluted in 250 ml. Give intravenously *only* at rate of 0.5 ml. per minute.
Caution: Severe skin and underlying tissue damage may result if extravasation occurs. (Rx - Regitine, see Chap. 2).

18. *Methylene blue:* 0.2 ml./kg. of 2% solution given I.V. over 5 minute period.

19. *Morphine sulfate:* Single dose: 0.1-0.2 ml./kg. Maximum dose: 15 mg. (1/4 grain).

20. *Paraldehyde:* 0.15 mg./kg. per dose, orally, rectally, or I.M.

21. *Phenergan:* 0.05 mg./kg. per dose.

22. *Phenobarbital:* SEDATION: 6 mg./kg. per 24 hours. Divide into 3 doses.

23. *Pyribenzamine:* 5 mg./kg. per 24 hours (maximum 150 mg.). Divide into 4-6 doses.

24. *Quinidine sulfate:* *Test* doses: 2 mg./kg.
Therapeutic dose: Children under 4 years: 30 mg./kg. per 24 hours. Children over 4 years: 200 mg. every 6-8 hours.

25. *Reserpine:* *For hypertension:* 0.07 *mg.*/kg. per 24 hours I.M. Give with apresoline 0.15 mg./kg. every 12-24 hours I.M.

26. *Thorazine:* a. 2.0 mg./kg. per 24 hours orally or I.M. Divide into 3-5 doses.
    b. Rectally, double the above dose.

B. ANTIMICROBIAL AGENTS

1. *Penicillin:*   Aqueous: *Infants:* 50,000 units/kg./ 24 hours.

Older children: 600,000 units/24 hours.

2. *Procaine:*　300,000-600,000 units per day I.M. in single dose.

3. *Bicillin:*　600,000-1.2 million units I.M. as a single dose.

CHAPTER 20

Treatment of Poisoning

IRA M. ROSENTHAL, M.D.

I. GENERAL CONSIDERATIONS

A. Poisonings constitute a significant portion of the medical emergencies faced by physicians. About 75% of the cases in the United States occur in children under 5 years of age. Poisoning is also common in retarded older children. Suicide and homicidal attempts also result in large numbers of poisonings. Occasional accidental ingestions are found in adults.

B. Household products such as bleaches, polishing fluids and pesticides are responsible for much of the poisoning in children. The medicine and kitchen cabinets are the usual sources of the poison. Studies at poison control centers throughout the United States have shown that over a thousand different products have been responsible.

C. In many cases, the diagnosis of poisoning is obvious and a history of ingestion is easily elicited. In some cases, it is difficult to elicit a history of ingestion or pica. In occasional cases, a history of ingestion is never obtained despite clinical and laboratory evidence for poisoning. In puzzling clinical problems in which the cause of the symptoms is not apparent, the possibility of poisoning should always be considered.

II. SIGNS, SYMPTOMS AND PHYSICAL FINDINGS

A. A large number of *symptoms* may develop as a result of poisoning. These include vomiting, pallor, convulsions, coma, somnolence, burning in the mouth, fever, collapse, hyperexcitability and diarrhea.

B. *Physical findings* suggestive of poisoning include disturbed states of consciousness, constricted pupils, dilated pupils, cyanosis, abnormal odor of tissues, increased sweating and alopecia. The urine may be discolored and the skin may be stained. The specific symptoms and physical findings often suggest the type of poison ingested.

III. IDENTIFICATION

A. Although the general nature of the poison may be indicated by symptoms and physical findings, definite identification of the agent is desirable. Examination of the original container from which the product was obtained is frequently helpful. As a result of the Federal Hazardous Substance Act, the containers of most dangerous household chemicals are labeled with a list of ingredients.

B. It must be recognized, however, that often the poisoning substance may *not* be in the original container but in a soda or milk bottle, a fruit jar or a drinking glass. Examination of the remainder of the tablets or pills from the container will often lead to identification of the poisoning compound.

C. A history of peeling paint or plaster at home or of other environmental hazards in the home, the industrial plant or a recreation site should also be elicited.

D. The toxicology laboratory is often helpful in the identification of the poisonous substance. Facilities for clinical toxicologic examination should be present in every hospital dealing with emergencies. Screening examinations for salicylates, barbiturates, diphenylhydantoin sodium (dilantin), glutethimide (Doriden) and amphetamines should be available locally. Arrangements should be made for referral of more difficult samples to a consulting or regional toxicology laboratory.

E. In dealing with cases of poisoning, appropriate tests of blood, urine, stomach contents or vomitus are useful.

In general, 10-20 ml. of clotted or heparinized blood, large volumes of urine such as 100 ml., if available, all stomach aspirants, all vomitus and the first lavage fluid should be sent to the laboratory. A chemically clean container should be used. The specimen should be *clearly labeled* with the name of the patient, the source of the specimen, the time the sample was collected, the condition of the patient and the name of the ward or emergency area and of the referring physician. Direct communication with the toxicology laboratory is helpful with regard to the test required and the urgency of the determination. If a specimen cannot be sent to the laboratory immediately, it should be refrigerated. "Preservatives" should not be added.

F. Nonspecific examinations such as hemoglobin and hematocrit tests for anemia, determinations for methemoglobinemia and urine coproporphyrin may be of value in the assessment of cases of poisoning.

IV. ATTEMPTED SUICIDES

A. Suicidal attempts utilizing the ingestion of poisonous substances or excessive doses of medications are common. There is a high frequency in adolescent and post-adolescent girls as well as in older depressed individuals. About 50% of adult ingestions are the result of attempts at suicide.

B. In addition to treatment for the poisoning, attention *must* be given to the psychiatric problems underlying the suicide attempt. Hospitalization is desirable in many such cases. Psychiatric evaluation is essential after the patient has recovered from the immediate effects of the ingestion. If there is suspicion of a *homicidal* attempt, appropriate *legal* authorities must be notified. The possibility of child abuse must also be considered.

V. PRINCIPLES OF MANAGEMENT

A. In the management of poisoning, *three main principles* are:

1. The poison should be evacuated or its absorption inhibited, if this can be done with safety.
2. Supportive and symptomatic therapy should be instituted promptly including administration of intravenous fluids and maintenance of an adequate airway.
3. If there is a specific antidote for the poison ingested, it should be administered. However, in only a small percentage of poisonings are specific antidotes known. The availability of a specific antidote does not obviate the need for general supportive measures.

B. Early in the evaluation of each case a decision must be made with regard to the necessity for hospitalization. All ingestions do not require hospitalization. In doubtful cases, however, hospitalization is mandatory because of possible medical-legal problems.

C. In dealing with ingestions, a prime consideration is whether *evacuation* of the stomach is indicated either by the induction of *vomiting* or by *gastric lavage*. It must be remembered that evacuation of the stomach is *contraindicated* in poisonings caused by corrosives such as lye or strong acids. Evacuation is *also contraindicated* if aspiration of small amounts of the poisonous substance is likely to cause *severe aspiration pneumonia*. Among such substances are kerosene, furniture polish and other petroleum products. Massive ingestion of one of these compounds may call for an occasional exception to the general rule of nonevacuation of these products. It has also been suggested that gastric lavage not be done after strychnine or glutethimide ingestion because of the danger of inducing convulsions or larynogospasm.

1. In most cases the induction of vomiting for emptying the stomach in cases of poisoning is more efficacious and faster than gastric lavage. Induction of vomiting should *not* be attempted, however, in unconscious or stuporous individuals. Although vomiting may be induced in a child with a finger or a spoon, the *preferred* method is ingestion of *syrup* of

ipeca. In fact, a 30-ml. bottle of this medication
should be in every household with small children.

2. The initial dose is 15 ml., and the medication should
be followed by ingestion of about 200 ml. of water
or clear fluids. Vomiting usually occurs within 20
minutes. If vomiting does not occur, the dose may
be repeated once. A slightly smaller dose should be
used in children under 1 year of age. Syrup of
ipecac is *contraindicated* after phenothiazine poisoning because of the antimetic properties of these compounds.

3. Gastric *lavage* can be employed in unconscious or
stuporous patients or if induction of vomiting with
syrup of ipecac is not successful. Gastric lavage is
contraindicated after ingestion of caustics, ammonia,
strychnine and most petroleum products. Children
should be restrained for lavage with the head slightly
dependent and the face turned to one side. A lubricated large bore catheter (greater than 28 French)
should be employed. Physiologic saline can be employed for lavage with instillation and subsequent
aspiration of 200-ml. amounts of the fluid many
times until between 2-4 liters have been used.

D. ACTIVATED CHARCOAL

1. *Activated charcoal,* USP, (activated charcoal)
(Merck) (Norit, A. and Nuchar, C.) is useful in many
types of poisoning. It *adsorbs* many poisonous compounds and reduces absorption. Activated charcoal
should *not* be given with syrup of ipecac since it ab-
sorbs the latter. However, the charcoal may be giv-
en after vomiting has been induced.

2. Among the substances effectively bound by activated charcoal are aspirin, dextroamphetamine,
strychnine, chloraquine, dilantin, phenobarbital and
primaquine phosphate. Glutethemide is less effectively bound. Activated charcoal is of *no value* for
binding ethyl alcohol, methyl alcohol, caustic alkalis,
mineral acids, and organic phosphates.

3. The *dose* of activated charcoal is 2 or more table-spoons or 5 times the estimated dose of the poisonous substance. The charcoal is administered only once as soon as possible after the ingestion of the poisonous substance. Tap water is added to the activated charcoal to make a slurry. The material may then be administered by large spoon, glass or stomach tube. Aspiration should be avoided. Activated charcoal should be stored tightly sealed.

E. The list of poisonous substances which may be encountered is long. Reference books relating to poisons should be available in each hospital treating emergencies. Advice from a poison control center may be helpful in planning treatment.

VI. SPECIFIC POISONS

A. SALICYLATES

1. Salicylate poisoning commonly is encountered. It occurs in young children as a result of accidental ingestion, or from therapeutic overdosage. Salicylates are commonly used in suicide attempts particularly in adolescents. In young children, a respiratory or other primary illness may be complicated by secondary salicylate poisoning. Salicylates are *eliminated* primarily by conjugation with glycine to form salicyluric acid. Relative excretion tends to slow as the total amount of salicylates in the body increases. The delayed excretion is not related to availability of glycine.

2. *Symptoms* of salicylate poisoning include anorexia, fever, vomiting, sweating, flushed appearance, hyperventilation, delirium, coma and confulsions. A *history* of ingestion usually can be elicited. The *phenistix test* of urine is useful as is the ferric chloride test. *Plasma sodium* is usually normal but plasma *bicarbonate* is usually reduced as a result of hyperventilation. Reducing substances in the urine and ketonuria are common.

3. A blood salicylate level is very helpful. Levels above 35 mg./100 ml. are considered toxic although there is no good correlation between salicylate levels and symptoms. The level must be evaluated with consideration of the time elapsed since the ingestion.

4. **Treatment.**

    a. Vomiting should be induced by *syrup* of ipecac if ingestion has been relatively recent.

    b. I.V. fluids should be started. *Elevation of the urine pH* to above 7.5 is useful since the reabsorption of salicylate from urine is markedly *reduced* at alkaline pH and excretion of salicylate is greatly *enhanced* at alkaline pH. This form of treatment has been recommended by Whitten (Am. J. Dis. Child., 101:178, 1961). Winters, however, feels that rapid administration of sodium bicarbonate in such cases may be hazardous.

    c. In our experience, Whitten's therapy when used with salicylate levels over 30 mg./100 ml. with evidence of acidosis has been effective and safe. In this method, 18-36 mEq. of *sodium bicarbonate* is given I.V. over 5 minutes. If after 10 minutes, the urine is not alkaline an additional 15 mEq. is given I.V. and repeated each 10 minutes until the urine is alkaline. After the urine is alkaline, 9 mEq. of sodium bicarbonate per 100 ml. of 5% dextrose in one-third physiologic saline is given as a drip at 1.5-3.0 ml. per minute.

    d. After a good urinary flow is obtained, 30 mEq. of *potassium chloride* is added to each liter of I.V. fluid. Urine should be checked every 30 minutes and if acid another 13-18 mEq. of sodium bicarbonate should be given over a 5-minute period. An indwelling catheter is useful if there is difficulty collecting urine. After 2-5 hours of treatment, maintenance fluids may be started. In rare cases in which renal failure occurs hemodialysis or peritoneal dialysis may be considered.

B. LEAD POISONING

1. Lead poisoning occurs primarily among children 12-
    36 months of age who reside in urban areas. Hous-
    ing which is in a poor state of repair with old peel-
    ing paint which has a heavy lead concentration is
    associated with lead poisoning. A history of pica
    generally can be elicited. There is a seasonal inci-
    dence of lead poisoning. Most cases occur during
    the summer months.
2. *Symptoms* include vomiting, ataxia, change in per-
    sonality, anorexia, constipation, anemia, incoordi-
    nation, lethargy, apathy, convulsions and stupor.
3. The *diagnosis* may be difficult if there is no history
    of pica.
    a. Roentgenograms of the abdomen often reveal
        "lead lines," areas of increased density at the
        metaphyses.
    b. Anemia is usually present and basophilic stip-
        pling may be seen in erythrocytes in some cases.
    c. Coproporphyrin is found in the urine in most
        cases.
    d. The *best* test, however, for the diagnosis of lead
        poisoning is the whole blood lead level (not
        serum or plasma) done by atomic absorption
        spectrophotometer. A blood lead level above
        50 μg./100 ml. indicates significant exposure.
        A level above 75 μg./100 ml. indicates lead
        poisoning.
4. Rapid deterioration of children with lead poisoning
    may occur and *prompt treatment* is therefore essen-
    tial. Most children with lead poisoning should be
    hospitalized. Enemas should not be given.
    a. Urine flow is established by administration of
        10% dextrose in water in a dose of 10-20 ml./kg.
        over a period of 2 hours. Fluids are then con-
        tinued on a maintenance basis so that urine out-
        put ranges between 350-500 ml./m^2/day. Over-
        hydration is dangerous in lead poisoning and
        may induce seizures.

    b. Shortly after urinary flow is established, *BAL* (dimercaprol) is given in a dose of 4 mg./kg., I.M. Four hours later the dose of BAL is repeated and *edathamil calcium disodium (Ca EDTA)* in a dose of 12.5 mg./kg. is also given I.M. A small dose of procaine, added to the EDTA, will reduce local pain. BAL and EDTA are then administered every 4 hours for a period of 5 days. If *convulsions* occur, paraldehyde may be given I.M. in a dose of 0.3 ca./kg. with a maximal dose of 5 cc.

    c. If severe cerebral edema develops, mannitol, 20% solution, may be administered I.V. with an initial dose of 3 cc./kg.

    d. *Respiratory arrest* is a constant threat and preparations should be made for resuscitation and assisted respiration if this becomes necessary. Barbiturates and adrenocorticosteroids are contraindicated in lead poisoning.

C. IRON POISONING

  1. Iron poisoning is common in young children. Tablets containing iron, particularly ferrous sulphate, are often mistaken for candy by children. Occasionally poisoning may occur from liquid preparations containing iron.

  2. The *symptoms* include vomiting, pallor, diarrhea, and dehydration. Acidosis and shock may develop. A history of ingestion can usually be elicited.

  3. In the *management* of iron poisoning, the following measures are indicated.

    a. Syrup of ipecac should be administered to induce vomiting, even if vomiting has occurred before admission, to empty the stomach further.

    b. The stomach should *also be lavaged* with 1% sodium bicarbonate solution using a large bore stomach tube. Specimens of the vomitus or gastric aspirant (including partially broken-up tablets) should be sent to the toxicology laboratory.

c. Heparinized or clotted blood should be drawn on admission for serum iron and iron-binding capacity.

d. A "scout" film of the abdomen should be taken since iron-containing tablets are opaque and can often be seen in the roentgenogram.

e. Five grams of *Desferal mesylate* should be instilled into the stomach. The preparation used is the same as that which is employed for intravenous therapy. I.V. fluids should be started at once. One gram of Desferal mesylate should be given by slow I.V. drip at a rate not to exceed 15 mg./kg. per hour. In small infants, the dose should not be greater than 90 mg./kg. per day. The total amount of this dose should not be given in less than 6 hours. Each ampule of Desferal contains 500 mg. of lyophilized desferoxamine mesylate. This is prepared by dissolving the Desferal in 2 ml. of sterile water for injection. After the drug is in solution, it should be added to physiologic saline, 5% glucose in water or Ringer's lactate before administration. In severe cases, it may be necessary to continue Desferal every 6-12 hours by slow drip as described above. The total amount of the drug administered however should not exceed 6 Gm. Rarely, it may be necessary to continue therapy for as long as 72 hours.

f. Desferal can also be administered I.M. It is prepared by adding 2 ml. of sterile water for injection to each ampul of 500 mg. of lyophilized desferoxamine mesylate. One gram of this medication is administered I.M. and this is followed by 0.5 Gm. every 4 hours for 2 doses. Depending upon the clinical response, subsequent doses of 0.5 Gm. may be administered every 4-12 hours. The total amount should not exceed 6 Gm. in 24 hours. The I.M. route should not be used if the patient shows any signs of shock.

g. All *urine* should be collected and color change

after administration of Desferal should be noted.
A *red* color indicates heavy excretion of iron
and indicates that additional Desferal should be
given. If the urine does not change color or if it
returns to a normal color, therapy with Desferal
may be discontinued.

h. Symptomatic therapy should be carried out as
indicated. Occasionally treatment for shock is
necessary. The chelation therapy with Desferal
is only effective if there is good urinary output.
If severe oliguria or anuria should develop,
dialysis should be considered to remove the iron
chelate.

D. POISONING WITH KEROSENE AND RELATED HYDROCARBONS

1. Kerosene and other compounds containing hydro-
carbons are common causes of poisoning in young
children. Products frequently involved include
furniture polish, turpentine, lighter fluid and ben-
zene. A history of ingestion is usually elicited.
These children may develop pneumonia, pneumonitis and pulmonary edema.

2. *Symptoms* usually include choking and gagging,
cough, nausea, fever, weakness and central nervous
system depression. A chest roentgenogram may reveal pulmonary infiltration. Subsequently emphysema may develop.

3. **Treatment.**
   a. In this type of poisoning, syrup of ipecac should
   not be administered. Most authorities believe
   that gastric lavage in the usual case is also contraindicated since aspiration can occur and the incidence of pulmonary involvement is increased.
   If very large amounts of the hydrocarbon are ingested, lavage must be considered, despite its risk.
   Such patients must be hospitalized for observation.

   b. It may be necessary to utilize oxygen therapy,
   high humidity and I.V. fluids.

c. Adrenocorticosteroids have been employed in severe cases but their value is questionable.

E. LYE BURNS

1. Lye commonly is used in many households for cleaning drains and frequently is stored in a variety of receptacles including soda bottles. As such, it may be mistaken for the original edible material and ingested by small children. Most lye burns occur in children between 13 months and 5 years of age.

2. Burns may be noted on the lips, in the mouth, and in the throat. Excess salivation may be present. In such cases, the child should be hospitalized and observed. The great *threat* is the development of esophageal stenosis and stricture from an esophageal burn.

3. If an esophageal burn is suspected, adrenocorticosteroids should be started utilizing prednisone in a dose of 2 mg./kg./day. In severe cases, adrenocorticosteroids may have to be given parenterally in equivalent dosage. Intramuscular penicillin should also be administered.

4. Arrangement should be made for *esophagoscopy* to determine if a lye burn of the esophagus is present. The purpose of this examination is to determine if a burn is present, not to determine its extent. If no esophageal burn is present, the adrenocorticosteroids may be discontinued. If a lye burn is present, prednisone, 2 mg./kg./day or equivalent, is continued for 10 days and arrangements are made for early bouginage.

5. The management of ingestion of *ammonium hydroxide* and *permanganate* is essentially similar to that of lye. Household products such as "Chlorox" are frequently ingested by young children. However, such products practically never cause esophageal burns and in most cases esophagoscopy is not indicated.

F.   BARBITURATE POISONING

1.   Barbiturates are a common cause of poisoning. Ingestion is usually accidental in young children. Medications prescribed for epilepsy of another family member are frequently ingested by toddlers. In adolescents and older individuals, barbiturates are commonly employed in attempts at suicide.

2.   *Symptoms* of barbiturate poisoning include somnolence, stupor, contracted pupils, and, in severe cases, coma and respiratory depression. Hospitalization is indicated.

3.   An attempt should be made to *identify* the barbiturate which has been ingested by thin layer chromatography since the treatment for ingestion of long-acting barbiturates differs somewhat from that of intermediate barbiturates.

4.   In either case the *stomach* should be emptied at once. If the state of consciousness is depressed, gastric lavage should be employed.

5.   *Activated charcoal* should be administered since this reduces further absorption of the barbiturates.

6.   I.V. fluids should be used to maintain hydration and encourage urinary excretion of the drug.

7.   Great attention should be paid to maintenance of the *airway*. In severe cases, assisted respiration may be required.

8.   Alkaline diuresis can markedly increase the urinary excretion of the *long-acting* barbiturates such as phenobarbital. This type of therapy is much less effective for shorter acting barbiturates such as pentobarbital and secobarbital. Phenobarbital is not excessively bound to plasma protein and a considerable fraction of the drug is present in ionized form at alkaline pH. Sodium bicarbonate or sodium lactate may be used for alkalinization.

9.   In a small child, an attempt should be made to increase urinary excretion threefold.

10.   In adults, an attempt should be made to obtain excretion of as much as 10 liters of urine daily.

Mannitol, urea, ethacrynic acid or furosemide may be used to increase diuresis.

11. A *central venous catheter* is useful in severe cases to monitor venous pressure in the face of large amounts of I.V. fluid in order to avoid pulmonary edema or cardiac failure.

12. Adequate amounts of *sodium* and *potassium* should be given. *Calcium salts* are useful to avoid tetany in the face of alkalinization. The amount of sodium bicarbonate required is usually 2 mEq./kg. for the first 2 hours and between 3-4 mEq./kg. for 6-12 hours thereafter. The urine pH should be monitored.

13. *Pneumonia* frequently develops in patients with barbiturate poisoning and antibiotics should be administered only if this complication is suspected. Analeptics are contraindicated.

G. PROPOXYPHENE (DARVON) POISONING

1. Propoxyphene poisoning also produces depression. This drug is absorbed by activated charcoal which should be used after the stomach has been emptied.

2. Propoxyphene on occasion inhibits release of antidiuretic hormone and large volumes of urine may be excreted.

3. I.V. fluids may be required to maintain hydration. Since propoxyphene is often combined in medications with *acetanilid,* in ingestions of such mixtures, methemoglobinemia resulting from the acetanilid may complicate the clinical picture.

H. ORGANOPHOSPHATE POISONING

1. Organophosphates are commonly used as insecticides. These pesticides are a common and important cause of poisoning in children and adults. Among the organophosphates are malathion, parathion, TEPP and OMPA. These compounds may be ingested, inhaled or absorbed through the skin or eye. They inactivate acetylcholinesterase and cause accumulation of acetylcholine.

2. *Symptoms:* Blurred vision, headache, profuse sweating, abdominal cramping, nausea and vomiting. Respiratory distress, convulsions, cyanosis, shock or coma may develop.
3. *Physical examination:* Miosis is usually present although terminally mydriasis may develop.
4. Mental confusion is frequently found and muscular incoordination develops. *Areflexia* is usually present.
5. A history of exposure to an organophosphate pesticide 6 hours or less before the onset of symptoms can usually be elicited.
6. In the *diagnosis* of organophosphate poisoning, significant depression of cholinesterase activity in plasma and erythrocytes provides laboratory verification of the diagnosis. Heparinized blood (10 ml.) should be sent to the laboratory. Treatment, however, should not await the result of laboratory tests.
7. **Treatment.**
    a. Gastric lavage should be employed and a saline cathartic administered, if the pesticide has been ingested.
    b. Skin and clothing should be decontaminated.
    c. If there is *respiratory* difficulty, maintenance of an adequate airway is essential and assisted respiration may become necessary.
    d. Anticonvulsants such as thiopental sodium may be required.
8. A *specific antidote* for organophosphate poisoning is the administration of *atropine* I.V. The dose is 0.2 mg. for children under 2 years of age; 0.5 mg. for children 2-10 years of age and from 1-2 mg. for individuals over 10 years of age.

These large doses of atropine are well tolerated and should be administered I.V. The medication can be repeated every 10 minutes until signs of atropinization develop. The atropine, however, should *not* be given if cyanosis is present. After relief of cyanosis by appropriate respiratory measures, the atropine can be administered.

9. Pralidoxime (Protopam chloride) is also useful. This drug reactivates cholinesterase. Twenty-five to 50 mg./kg. in a 50% solution in isotonic saline can be given over a 5-10-minute period. It should be noted that Protopam is of questionable value 48 hours after exposure.

I. POISONING WITH PSYCHOACTIVE DRUGS

1. Poisoning with psychoactive drugs is becoming more common and is particularly prevalent among adolescents and young adults. *Four* groups of drugs are employed by such individuals. These are:
   a. Stimulants.
   b. Analeptics.
   c. Depressants or neuroleptics.
   d. Antidepressants or thymoleptics and consciousness-distorting drugs (dysleptic or psychedelic).
2. Cases of poisoning with psychoactive drugs are often difficult to diagnose and manage. These agents are frequently used in combination. It is very difficult to establish the drugs which have been used by history.
3. *Symptoms* include depression, hyperactivity, restlessness, seizures, and transient development of psychosis. In most cases conservative care is indicated.
   a. Dehydration should be avoided if possible and corrected if necessary.
   b. An adequate airway must be maintained.
   c. If severe restlessness is present, short-acting barbiturates such as pentobarbital or secobarbital in doses of 100 mg. may be used I.M. or I.V. Diazepam (Valium) in a dose of 5 mg. may be administered I.V. or I.M. Phenothiazines should be avoided because they are toxic after some of these agents and may precipitate excitement or hypertension.
4. *Heroin,* morphine, or codeine poisoning can be treated with appropriate narcotic antagonists such as nalorphine (Nalline). Reassurance is essential in the management of these patients.

5. In patients with *amphetamine* poisoning, acidification of the urine with forced diuresis is useful. Arginine monochloride, ascorbic acid or ammonium chloride may be given I.V.

6. *Methadone poisoning.* The introduction of methadone for the treatment of heroin addiction has resulted in occasional cases of accidental methadone poisoning in children.

    a. The *respiratory* status of the child suspected of methadone poisoning should be carefully assessed since death may result from respiratory depression.

    b. In addition to I.V. fluids and assisted respiration when indicated, administration of a narcotic antagonist is indicated in the face of respiratory depression or unconsciousness. Nalline, Lorfan or Narcan can be given I.V.

        1) Naloxone hydrochloride (Narcan) can be administered in a dose of 0.01 mg./kg., I.V.

        2) The dose of nalorphine hydrochloride (Nalline) is 0.1 mg./kg., I.V.

        3) The dose for levallorphan tartrate (Lorfan) is 0.02 mg./kg., I.V.

    c. It should be noted that if respiratory impairment is the result of barbiturate poisoning, respiration depression may be increased by Nalline and Lorfan. The action of these narcotic antagonists only lasts for 2-3 hours, and the depressant effect of methadone may persist for 48 hours.

    d. If respiration improves after the injection of the antagonist, a second injection can be given in 5 or 10 minutes. Repeated administration may be necessary to maintain respiration.

    e. If there is no improvement in respiration, additional doses of Nalline and Lorfan should be avoided. Repeated doses of the antagonist can be given I.M., but the dose is 50% greater than the I.V. dose.

    f. Dialysis and CNS stimulants are contraindicated.

g. Close observation of the patient is indicated until the effects of the poison have worn off.

7. *Acute alcoholism.*
    a. In the *management* of acute alcoholism, care
        must be taken as in many other forms of poison-
        ing to maintain an adequate airway. Rarely, as-
        sisted respiration is required.
    b. Dehydration sometimes induced by vomiting
        should be avoided or corrected by the use of I.V.
        fluids.
    c. Hypoglycemia may occur in individuals with
        acute alcoholism, particularly in young children,
        and must be treated vigorously with glucose so-
        lutions administered I.V.

8. *Methanol poisoning.*
    a. The laboratory should be able to detect metha-
        nol in a blood sample. Methanol can cause se-
        vere central nervous system depression. In addi-
        tion, ingestion of methanol can result in blind-
        ness. Methanol is converted to form formalde-
        hyde and formic acid. Formaldehyde can cause
        blindness and formic acid severe acidosis.
    b. In the *management* of methanol poisoning, alkali
        therapy may be necessary.
    c. *Ethanol* may be employed as a competitive in-
        hibitor. Ethanol has a higher affinity for alcohol
        dehydrogenase than methanol, and formation of
        formaldehyde and formic acid is reduced.
    d. The dose of ethanol is 1 oz. of 80 proof whiskey
        at hourly intervals to maintain a blood alcohol
        level between 70 and 100 mg./100 ml.

J. PHENOTHIAZINE POISONING

1. Phenothiazine poisoning is common and may devel-
    op as a result of excessive ingestion of these medica-
    tions or as a result of hypersensitivity to these drugs.
2. *Symptoms* include abnormal movements, oculogyric
    crisis, neck retraction, torticollis, flexor rigidity, and
    hyperreflexia.

3. **Treatment.** Gastric lavage is indicated. Administration of syrup of ipecac is *contraindicated* since most of the phenothiazines are antiemetic drugs.
   a. In the treatment of the extrapyramidal symptoms, *diphenhydramine hydrochloride* (benadryl hydrochloride) is frequently of value. The *dose* employed is 50 mg. I.V. over a period of 5 minutes.
   b. The FPN reagent is useful for screening urine for phenothíazine poisoning.

K. MERCURY POISONING

1. Metallic mercury is not absorbed and does not cause mercury poisoning. *Mercury salts,* however, are extremely toxic. Poisoning may occur with mercury bichloride tablets or excessive amounts of calomel or ammoniated mercury.
2. *Symptoms.* Throat and esophageal lesions develop and there may be abdominal pain, vomiting, bloody diarrhea, and signs of renal failure.
3. **Therapy** includes copious lavage after a protein-containing food such as milk or raw egg has been introduced into the stomach.
   a. Fifteen to 30 ml. of magnesium sulfate may be administered in 6 oz. of milk.
   b. The *major* therapy, however, is BAL (dimercaprol) which is administered in a dose of 3 mg./kg. every 4 hours x 6 for a 2-day period, then in a dose of 3 mg./kg. every 6 hours x 4 doses, and subsequently in a dose of 3 mg./kg. every 12 hours x 2 days. In less severe cases a smaller dose may be used.
   c. Urinalysis should be performed daily and the blood urea nitrogen followed.

L. RODENTICIDES

The most common rodenticide ingested is Warfarin. This compound is not very toxic to humans and will only produce hypoprothrombinemia after repeated administration. In most cases, therapy after ingestion is not necessary, although vitamin K may be administered.

REFERENCES

1. Gleason, M. N., Gosselin, R. E., Hodge, H. C., and Smith, R. P.: *Clinical Toxicology of Commercial Products: Acute Poisoning* (3d ed.; Baltimore: Williams & Wilkins, 1969).

2. Goodman, L. S., and Gilman, A., eds.: *The Pharmacological Basis of Therapeutics:* A Textbook of Pharmacology, Toxicology, and Therapeutics for Physicians and Medical Students (4th ed.; New York: Macmillan Co., 1970).

3. Arena, J. M.: *Poisoning: Chemistry, Symptoms, Treatments* (Springfield, Ill.: Charles C Thomas, Publisher, 1963).

4. Deichmann, W. B., and Gerarde, H. W. S.: *Toxicology of Drugs and Chemicals* (New York, London: Academic Press, Inc., 1969).

CHAPTER 21

Pediatric Surgical Emergencies

JOHN G. RAFFENSPERGER, M.D.

The pediatric surgeon's job is to save life and restore function, but he must not produce fear and insecurity through indifferent or thoughtless handling of a child. The child's emotional makeup must be considered. In an emergency, take the parents into your confidence and explain the projected procedure. Secure their cooperation in the preoperative and postoperative periods.

I. NEWBORN SURGICAL EMERGENCIES

Some of the most important emergencies are those in the newborn period. Specific preoperative and postoperative care depends on the individual baby, but, in general, the following apply to all newborn surgical problems:

1. Temperature control.
2. Humidity.
3. Oxygen.
4. Antibiotics.
5. 0.5 to 1 mg. of vitamin K.
6. Gastric tube.
7. Nasopharyngeal suction.
8. Type and cross match.
9. Upper extremity cutdown.

The first three needs are met by a warm, humidified incubator. Provisions for warmth must be made during x-ray studies, transportation and while doing procedures such as cutdowns. The need for antibiotics can be debated but, in infants with respiratory distress or where opening of the intestine is anticipated, they should be used. We prefer ampicillin and 10 mg./kg. per day of kanamycin in 2 divided doses.

A. RESPIRATORY DISTRESS

Diagnostic studies of the infant with respiratory distress commence with observations of the respiratory rate, pulse, location of the apex beat and careful auscultation for diminished breath sounds. At the bedside one can pass a catheter through the nose and into the stomach to check for obstruction. Palpate the oropharynx, then inspect the vocal cords with a laryngoscope. Good PA and lateral chest x-ray films are essential and often a lipiodol study of the esophagus is necessary to discover esophageal abnormalities or vascular rings.

B. OBSTRUCTIVE LESIONS

1. Choanal atresia should be considered when the infant gasps for air, and remains cyanotic until he opens his mouth and cries. The diagnosis is made when one cannot pass a catheter through the nose. In an emergency, pull the tongue forward and insert an oral airway. A tracheotomy may be necessary until the choanal atresia can be dealt with.
2. The Pierre-Robin syndrome consists of a small mandible and a midline cleft palate; often the tongue falls back against the pharynx. Treatment consists of keeping the child in the prone position and insertion of a nasogastric feeding tube. A tongue traction suture or a tracheostomy occasionally is necessary.
3. The thyroglossal duct cyst at the base of the tongue may cause almost complete airway obstruction. The diagnosis is made by palpation of the lingual mass. The cyst can be first aspirated then marsupialized.
4. Vascular rings such as a double aortic arch rarely cause significant airway obstruction in the early newborn period. They may be suspected when there are repeated bouts of wheezing and frequent upper respiratory infections. The diagnosis is made by the

indentation on the back wall of the esophagus, on a barium esophagogram.

C. LESIONS WHICH DISPLACE PULMONARY TISSUE

1. Diaphragmatic hernia should be considered in an infant with cyanosis, tachypnea and a scaphoid abdomen. Most commonly, the hernia is through the left foramen of Bochdalek, so there are no breath sounds in the left chest and the heart is shifted to the right (Fig. 21-1). A chest x-ray film outlines intestine in the thorax. Surgical treatment should be immediate; the abdominal approach is preferred. Often, after the intestine has been withdrawn from the chest, it will not be possible to close the abdominal peritoneum and fascia because the intestine has lost its right of domicile. Preoperative and postoperative oxygen therapy in an incubator is essential. The blood Pco_2, Po_2 and pH should be determined before and after operation. Sodium bicarbonate and buffers are often necessary to correct severe respiratory acidosis.

Fig. 21-1.–Diaphragmatic hernia.

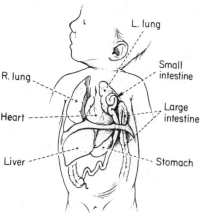

2. Pneumothorax is often found in infants who require vigorous resuscitation. If the lung is compressed and the mediastinum is shifted, insert a size 10 or 12 catheter in the pleural cavity in the midaxillary line and connect it to a water seal. The lung should expand promptly, and if there is no air leakage, the tube can be removed in 24 hours.

D. ESOPHAGEAL ATRESIA AND TRACHEOESOPHAGEAL FISTULA

1. Hypersalivation, choking on feedings, and respiratory distress are symptomatic of esophageal anomalies. The diagnosis is easily made by passing a catheter through the nose and injecting 1/2 ml. of lipiodol. An x-ray film will then show the esophageal atresia. If there is air in the gastrointestinal tract, a fistula is present. Figure 21-2 diagrams the three most common anomalies.

Fig. 21-2. –Esophageal malformations.

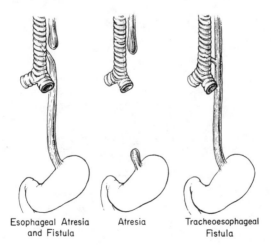

Esophageal Atresia   Atresia   Tracheoesophageal
and Fistula   Fistula

2. Infants with an atresia and fistula aspirate gastric juice as well as saliva into the lungs. They develop atelectasis and pneumonia unless the diagnosis is made promptly. Therapy consists of frequent aspiration of the airway, with a laryngoscope if necessary. Oxygen, humidity, and antibiotics are routinely administered. Operation can be delayed until the lungs are clear. A gastrostomy performed under local anesthesia will reduce gastric reflux prior to the definitive repair. In a poor-risk infant, the esophageal anastomosis can be delayed several days after the gastrostomy to give the infant time to clear pneumonia and atelectasis. Infants with an atresia and no fistula often have only a short nubbin of distal esophagus. Consequently, all that is done is a cervical esophagostomy and a gastrostomy. Later, a colon by-pass restores esophageal continuity (Fig. 21-3). Type 3 or the H fistula is difficult to diagnose, but should be suspected in infants with repeated bouts of pneumonia, aspiration, and abdominal distention. The cine-esophagram or direct examination of the trachea with a bronchoscope offers the best chance for diagnosis.

Fig. 21-3. –Stages in therapy of esophageal atresia.

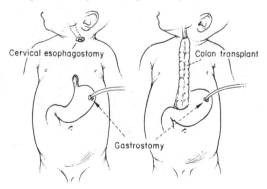

Cervical esophagostomy

Colon transplant

Gastrostomy

E. CONGENITAL HEART DISEASE

Infants who have cyanosis but no significant respiratory distress are likely to have a right-to-left intracardiac shunt. On the other hand, babies with large left-to-right shunts through a patent ductus or a large ventricular septal defect may have severe tachypnea and tachycardia as well as an enlarged liver, and are often thought to have pneumonia rather than congenital heart disease. This is because more than 50% of infants with anomalies of the heart have no murmurs during the first few days. Consequently, palpate all pulses, repeatedly examine the chest and have serial x-ray films for heart size and an electrocardiogram on all children with undiagnosed respiratory distress.

F. INTESTINAL OBSTRUCTION (Fig. 21-4)

1. There are three cardinal signs of intestinal obstruction in newborn infants.
    a. *Green* or biliary vomiting.
    b. Abdominal distention.
    c. Failure to pass a meconium stool in the first 24 hours of life.
2. Any one of these symptoms demands the immediate insertion of a nasogastric tube to prevent vomiting and aspiration and an upright roentgenogram of the abdomen. The diagnosis of almost all newborn intestinal obstructions can be made with this single x-ray film. Atresias of the duodenum and small intestine are recognized by air fluid levels in the bowel. Treatment consists of decompression of the stomach by a nasogastric tube and fluid and electrolyte replacement. If the infant is severely dehydrated, plasma is indicated to correct deficiencies in blood volume. Proximal atresias are treated by resection and anastomosis of the atretic intestine, while atresia of the ileum may be either resected and immediately anastomosed or exteriorized.

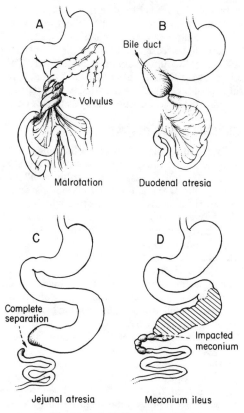

Fig. 21-4.—Intestinal obstruction.

G. MALROTATION OF THE MIDGUT

This entity usually presents in the first week of life with biliary vomiting. The obstruction usually is only partial and a barium swallow may be necessary if the plain films are not diagnostic. A midgut volvulus accompanies malrotation and if there is blood in the stool, operation is urgently needed to prevent gangrene. Treatment consists of gastric decompression, fluids and electrolytes and the Ladd operation; adhesions from the colon to the lateral abdominal wall which cross the duodenum must be severed. This frees the cecum to lie on the left side of the abdomen. The midgut volvulus is reduced and a gastrostomy is performed to prevent gastric distention in the postoperative period.

H. HIRSCHSPRUNG'S DISEASE

1. Hirschsprung's disease is suspected when a baby is distended and must have an enema or rectal examination to secure passage of meconium. Plain roentgenograms of the abdomen will demonstrate multiple air fluid levels in the intestine which may be confused with an atresia of the ileum. Consequently, a barium enema is in order to find the distal narrow colon; a biopsy of the rectal wall will establish the absence of ganglion cells.

2. Untreated Hirschsprung's disease in the newborn carries a mortality as high as 50% because of enterocolitis and sepsis; consequently, a colostomy at the distal limit of colon containing ganglion cells is indicated (Fig. 21-5).

3. A pull-through operation is then done at 6-9 months of age.

4. In the postoperative period, after repair of an intestinal obstruction, there may be a prolonged paralytic ileus. During this time, fluids and electrolytes must be carefully replaced and maintained. The stomach must be constantly emptied with a gastrostomy or nasogastric tube; serial body weights, serum electrolytes and frequent clinical examinations are necessary to guide replacement fluid therapy. Overhydration is prevented by giving only enough fluids so that the baby loses approximately 15 Gm. per day.

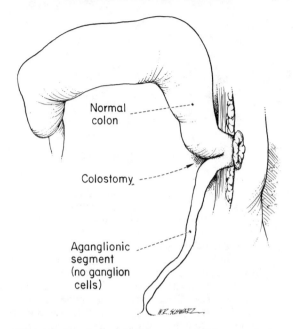

Fig. 21-5.—Hirschsprung's disease (congenital megacolon).

I.   IMPERFORATE ANUS (Fig. 21-6)

1.   Female infants will almost always have a rectoperi-
     neal or rectal vaginal fistula associated with imper-
     forate anus. If the fistula is not readily apparent,
     carefully separate the labia and examine the vagina
     with a nasal speculum and a good light. Ectopic
     anus may be a better term for this anomaly in girls
     because often the fistula will function perfectly
     well, and the surgical repair can be delayed for sev-
     eral months. A perineal anoplasty is successful in
     restoring the anus to its normal position, and anal
     function in female infants is always excellent after
     a good repair.

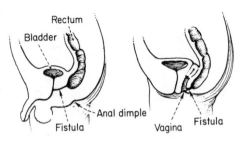

Fig. 21-6.–Imperforate anus.

2. Males with an imperforate anus have an entirely different problem. The rectal pouch usually lies 2½-3 cm. from the perineal skin and there is a fistula to the bladder or to the urethra. For this reason, a microscopic urinalysis is performed to detect meconium, and an x-ray film is taken with the infant inverted, with a small lead marker held in the anal dimple (Wangensteen-Rice technique). The distance from the gas-filled rectum to the marker is measured. If it is less than 1.5 cm., it may be possible to repair the defect through a perineal incision. When the distance is more than 1.5 cm., and when there is a fistula to the urinary tract, a combined abdomino-perineal operation will be necessary. A completely diverting sigmoid colostomy is the safest procedure in the newborn. Then a very careful sphincter-saving operation can be done at 9 months to 1 year of age.

J. OMPHALOCELE

1. Small umbilical defects may be operated on immediately and completely closed with good results. Large omphaloceles which contain liver and small intestine are difficult to repair because if all of the viscera is forced back into the abdomen, the diaphragms are elevated and respiratory distress results. Consequently, no attempt is made to close the fascia, but skin is

mobilized and closed over the sac. Even this procedure is dangerous and carries a high mortality
rate. Recently, attempts have been made to merely
paint the sac with 1% mercurochrome until it
shrinks down and becomes covered with epithelium.

2. If an infant has one congenital defect, he is likely to
have another. Commonly associated lesions are imperforate anus with tracheoesophageal fistula, duodenal atresia with mongolism, malrotation with
diaphragmatic hernias and omphaloceles, and geni-
tourinary disease with Hirschsprung's disease and
an imperforate anus.

3. A newborn baby with a congenital defect needs the
best in pediatric and surgical care to survive. The
result is a 70-year cure.

II. SURGICAL CONDITIONS IN OLDER CHILDREN

A. PYLORIC STENOSIS

Characteristically, pyloric stenosis occurs at the age
of 2-6 weeks in the first-born male infant, and the
vomiting is described as projectile. However, do not
forget that pyloric stenosis can occur in an infant from
1 week to several months of age and may occur in girls
as well as in boys. The initial vomiting may not be projectile, and the infant who has been weakened with prolonged vomiting and malnutrition may only drool out
the side of his mouth and be too weak to forcefully
vomit. Any infant seen as an outpatient who is vomiting and who has lost weight should be hospitalized for
investigation. Physical examination starts with the
fontaneles to determine the degree of dehydration, or
to find bulging. Sit down beside the infant, feed him
and watch for peristaltic waves. Palpate the abdomen
only when the infant is completely relaxed, preferably
immediately after a vomiting episode. The pyloric
mass is elusive and may be located anywhere from the
midepigastrium to the right upper quadrant tucked under the liver. X-ray films of the stomach with contrast

material are not necessary to diagnose pyloric stenosis if the mass is present and they may be potentially harmful because vomiting and aspiration is the most common cause of death in these infants. If an experienced examiner cannot find the mass on repeated examination, x-ray films should be made with attention to the esophagus to detect chalasia or a sliding hiatus hernia, which may simulate pyloric stenosis. When the diagnosis of pyloric stenosis has been made, the stomach is emptied with a size 12 nasogastric tube and irrigated to remove all curded milk. The tube is then left on gravity drainage. Electrolytes can be restored in 12-24 hours with 1/2 normal saline plus 40 mEq. of potassium chloride per liter. When fluids and electrolytes have been restored toward normal, the classic Ramstedt pyloromyotomy may be done under local or general anesthesia. Some surgeons feed these infants within the first 4 hours. It is safer to wait 12-24 hours.

B. INTUSSUSCEPTION

Intussusception occurs commonly in infants at approximately 6 months of age. The mother will note that the child pulls his knees up to his abdomen, cries with pain and then relaxes. These paroxysms occur 15-20 minutes apart and the child may sleep in the interval. Vomiting is common and a stool mixed with blood and mucus is often passed during the first 12 hours of this illness. If the infant is seen prior to the development of abdominal distention, a sausage-shaped mass may be palpated in the abdomen. If upright films of the abdomen reveal air fluid levels diagnostic of an intestinal obstruction, attention should be directed to treatment of shock, replacement of fluids and an early operation. On the other hand, if the abdomen is not distended or tender, and if the child is seen during the first 24 hours, a barium enema should be performed to reduce the intussusception. Hydrostatic pressure is popular and safe, as it carries a lower morbidity and mortality than operation. The surgeon should be present during the barium enema reduction and the barium container should never be held more than 3 feet above the level of the patient. Complete reduction is signaled by passage of the barium into the terminal ileum. Following an apparently successful reduction, the child should fall asleep and have no more episodes of crampy abdominal pain. If signs of obstruction persist, an operation should be performed to complete the reduction of the intussusception.

C. INCARCERATED HERNIA

Hernias are common in children under 1 year of age. They should be repaired when the diagnosis is made, provided the child is in good general condition. When a child is admitted with a swollen, tender scrotum in which the diagnosis could be incarcerated hernia, sedate him, put him in the Trendelenburg position, but do not push on the scrotal mass. Insert a nasogastric tube and replace fluid and electrolytes if he has vomited. Surgical repair is performed if the hernia does not reduce spontaneously in 1 to 2 hours.

D. TORSION OF THE TESTICLE

Torsion of the testicle is not uncommon in children and may be suspected when an infant cries out suddenly and is found to have a swollen testicle. Operation must be performed within 6 hours if the testicle is to be salvaged. At the time of operation, the testicle is untwisted and the tunica albuginea is incised. Apply ice bags to the scrotum in the postoperative period. An orchiectomy should never be done! Since this can occur bilaterally, the opposite testicle is attached to the tunica vaginalis with 2 or 3 sutures.

E. GASTROINTESTINAL BLEEDING

In the newborn period, small amounts of blood may be vomited or passed in the stool secondary to the ingestion of maternal blood or in hypoprothrombinemia. Close observation, gastric lavage and treatment with vitamin K is usually all that is indicated. Occasionally, fresh whole blood is necessary to replace blood volume and clotting factors. In older infants, anal fissures cause blood streaking in the stool. A history of the passage of a hard stool with crying is obtained. Place the infant in the prone position and retract the buttocks to see the fissure. Treatment consists of stool softeners, local application of soothing ointments and reassurance to the parents.

F. COLON POLYPS

1. Polyps in children rarely cause pain or severe hemorrhage. A small amount of blood is found on the surface of the stool. Seventy-five per cent of rectal polyps are within reach of the palpating finger or proctoscope, but an air contrast barium enema may be necessary to find polyps higher in the colon. Remove polyps within reach of the proctoscope with a snare and cautery. Polyps higher in the colon need not be treated, since these are inflammatory lesions and never become malignant. If bleeding is severe enough to cause anemia, these polyps may be removed by laparotomy and colotomy.

2. Massive gastrointestinal hemorrhage should prompt the immediate insertion of a Levin tube to determine whether blood is originating from the stomach or lower intestinal tract. Esophageal varices and duodenal ulcers can bleed massively, causing bright red blood to appear in the stools because of increased peristalsis. After insertion of the nasogastric tube, stabilize the child's blood volume with transfusions and then proceed with gastrointestinal x-ray films, looking for esophageal varices or a duodenal ulcer.

3. Esophageal varices in a child may be treated with a Blakemore tube and blood transfusions until the immediate hemorrhage has passed. A shunting operation is then performed at a later date.

4. Bleeding from a duodenal ulcer will usually cease

spontaneously in older children. However, if the
duodenal ulcer accompanies another disease, such
as burns or central nervous system lesions, operation
is indicated when the child has lost the equivalent
of his own blood volume.

5. A Meckel's diverticulum is suspected when no
other source of lower intestinal bleeding is identified.

6. Bleeding from a Meckel's diverticulum usually will
stop spontaneously, but a transfusion is indicated
for shock or a hemoglobin level below 6 Gm. A
laparotomy is the only way to establish the diagnosis of a Meckel's diverticulum, but operation
is usually delayed until the second significant episode.

G. APPENDICITIS

1. Appendicitis is always included in the differential
diagnosis when a child has abdominal pain. If the
pain is at first vague and diffuse, then settles in the
right lower quadrant, the diagnosis can almost be
made by history alone. Anorexia, nausea, vomiting
and constipation are usually, but not always, present. When you examine a child with suspected appendicitis, spend a few minutes talking to him, tell
him a story and warm your hands before you touch
him. During this time, observe his face and position
in bed. If he looks worried and lies very still, he is
likely to have intraperitoneal inflammation. Palpate
superficially, first at the left iliac crest, then gently
over the entire abdomen, while watching his face for
a frown or a wince. Deeper palpation is then carried out, but avoid sudden movements or surprising,
painful manipulations such as the test for rebound
tenderness. It is often helpful to have the child
poke with his finger to find his own sore spot. If
deep pressure in the left lower quadrant elicits right-
sided pain, and if there is persistent right lower quadrant tenderness, the diagnosis is assured. A retrocecal

appendix may simulate pyelonephritis, and the abdominal findings may be minimal. Also, if the appendix is deep in the pelvis, the child will have only rectal tenderness. Repeated examinations, particularly by an experienced surgeon, is the best diagnostic measure, but the white blood count and the microscopic urinalysis may help.

2. Appendicitis in young children is a rapidly progressive disease which can go on to peritonitis and severe toxicity in a few hours. You must replace fluid lost by vomiting and that sequestered in loops of intestine before the operation. Febrile convulsions may complicate the anesthetic unless the temperature is reduced to 100° or less with rectal aspirin, external hypothermia and chlorpromazine before the child is taken to the Operating Room. Many diseases cause abdominal pain in childhood which mimic acute appendicitis. The common offenders include acute pharyngitis with viral enteritis, acute pyelonephritis and the "green apple bellyache." If you keep in mind lead poisoning, diabetic acidosis, pneumonia, acute rheumatic fever and the allergic purpuras and meningitis, you are not likely to make the error of performing an appendectomy on a child with a serious medical disease. Mesenteric adenitis is a diagnosis made by surgeons after they remove a normal appendix!

3. After an operation for a perforated appendix, remain alert for a persistent fever and the signs of a subphrenic or pelvic abscess. Do not make the mistake of treating the fever with changes of antibiotics while an abscess smolders along, becoming larger every day.

4. Today, one of the worst medical tragedies occurs when a child with an atypical appendicitis is sent home from a hospital Emergency Room or from a physician's office. You had better err on the side of an occasional unnecessary admission to the hospital of a child with abdominal pain than run the risk of missing the diagnosis completely.

H. FOREIGN BODIES IN THE GASTROINTESTINAL TRACT

1. A child's normal learning process includes the testing of various objects for taste and consistency in the mouth. Some of these things are swallowed. Most are small enough to pass through without difficulty, but some stay in the esophagus or the stomach.

2. If a foreign body lodges in the esophagus, the child will hypersalivate and refuse to swallow. Metallic objects are seen on a plain roentgenogram, but others require a swallow of lipiodol or barium to outline the object. Esophagoscopic removal is indicated for all foreign objects in the esophagus when the child is afebrile and well hydrated. More than 90% of foreign bodies which reach the stomach uneventfully go through the remainder of the intestine. Children with coins or other round objects in the stomach or intestine are admonished not to swallow similar articles and their parents are advised to watch the stools and to bring the child back if there is any trouble. Children who have ingested such sharp objects as an open safety pin, needles or a bobby pin need close observation and repeated roentgen examinations. If the object remains in one place for 5 days, particularly in the duodenal curve, suspect a perforation of the bowel wall. An operation to remove the object is then indicated.

I. ABDOMINAL TRAUMA IN CHILDREN

1. Evaluate an injured child rapidly, but as systematically as if you were doing a complete medical workup! During the first few minutes, you should *establish the airway,* if this is compromised, evaluate the *level of consciousness* and note the *vital signs;* then commence palpation at the head, check for cervical tenderness or instability, passively move and palpate the extremities, compress the pelvis, then look at the abdomen. Injuries in other areas of the body

are usually found by the simple rapid maneuvers described above, but intra-abdominal injury may become evident only after repeated examinations and serial laboratory determinations. Acute gastric distention and paralytic ileus usually point to some intra-abdominal problems, but may be secondary to trauma elsewhere. However, if there is any suspicion of an intra-abdominal injury, based on an obvious superficial bruise, tenderness, distention, an unexplained rapid pulse, hematuria or only abdominal pain, the following procedures are carried out: A needle is inserted into a vein and blood is drawn for a hematocrit and a type and crossmatch, then lactated Ringer's solution is started through the same needle. A Levin tube is inserted and the stomach lavaged, particularly if there has been a recent meal. If the child can void, the urine is examined for red blood cells; if not, a urethral catheter is inserted. If further therapy is needed at this time, such as a blood transfusion, it is started, then the child is taken to the X-ray Department. Remember to splint fractures and to make all transfers from stretchers to the x-ray table as atraumatic as possible. The responsible surgeon accompanies the child to interpret the films and to determine the need for additional roentgenograms. Flat and upright films of the abdomen and chest are always obtained; in addition, if there is hematuria or flank tenderness, an intravenous pyelogram is performed. If there is a fracture of the pelvis, a cystourethrogram is essential to rule out injuries to the urethra and bladder.

2. Often an evaluation of the physical findings, roentgenograms and the hematocrit will indicate that an exploratory laparotomy is indicated. On the other hand, if the findings are equivocal or if there are other injuries which may increase the risk of anesthesia and an exploratory operation, an abdominal paracentesis is indicated. A negative tap is meaningless but, if nonclotted blood on free fluid is obtained, an operation is indicated. To perform an abdominal

tap on a child, have him lie on his side and prepare an area in the lower quadrant on the dependent side. The skin and abdominal wall are infiltrated with a local anesthetic, using a 25-gauge needle to minimize pain and apprehension. A 20-gauge needle is then gently inserted until the peritoneum is felt to "give."

3. If there is a suggestion of an abdominal injury, and the surgeon cannot definitely make up his mind, the child is critically re-evaluated at hourly intervals, with serial hematocrits and more roentgenograms, if necessary. During the period of observation, other injuries are treated and a nasogastric tube is left in place to ensure that the stomach will be empty if an operation does become necessary.

4. This approach to abdominal trauma in children will assure that delayed ruptures of the spleen are detected and that the subtle signs of a retroperitoneal injury of the duodenum will not be overlooked. Before the child is taken to the Operating Room with an obvious intra-abdominal injury, make certain that the urinary catheter and Levin tube are functioning. A central venous pressure catheter is helpful to evaluate blood losses and at least 2000 ml. of blood should be typed, crossmatched and in the Operating Room.

CHAPTER 22

Pediatric Anesthesia in the Emergency Service

REUBEN C. BALAGOT, M.D., *and*
VALERIE R. BANDELIN, M.D.

I. INTRODUCTION

Emergency pediatric general anesthesia is essentially outpatient pediatric anesthesia. The main difference lies in that the pediatric patient is totally unprepared for surgery. Mitigation of the problems can simplify to some extent the anesthetic management. Inability to do so increases the complexity and may make the simplest case unmanageable or very difficult.

Due to the urgency of the situation, the opportunity of preparing the patient properly is greatly reduced. It is rare that the patient has an empty stomach. Should general anesthesia be necessary, vomiting and aspiration may occur. There are maneuvers for diminishing these hazards, but the possibility remains. A preoperative enema is not helpful, however.

Any and every patient receiving a general anesthetic should be:

1. In the *main* operating rooms, if possible.
2. Be *admitted* to the *hospital* after the procedure, if at all possible.

II. PREOPERATIVE MEDICATION

Considering the urgency of the situation, having the patient well sedated, emotionally stable and protected from overactivity of the autonomic nervous system is not easily achieved.

The belladonna drugs, the shorter acting narcotic analgesics and possibly the barbiturates are helpful.

A. BELLADONNA DRUGS

1. If circumstances do not warrant the administration of sedative and tranquilizing drugs, the one single premedicant drug that almost any anesthesiologist would use is *atropine* or *scopolamine*. The main objective is to dry up secretions in the oropharyngeal area and the tracheobronchial tree and somehow mitigate the general anesthetic complications referable to the parasympathetic system.

2. From the secretion-drying aspect, *scopolamine* is much superior to *atropine*. However, from the point of view of vagal blockade, atropine easily surpasses scopolamine, and may be an advantage. Scopolamine has one other advantage over atropine, and that is its ability to cause some amount of sedation and amnesia. In children, particularly in an emergency situation, the sedation afforded by scopolamine enables one to avoid the use of barbiturates or narcotics, both of which can cause respiratory depression. Depression from the narcotic and complications from the barbiturate can be reversed, but it is decidedly advantageous for the outpatient, after leaving the operative room to have as little depression of vital functions as possible.

3. *Dosage.* —It is always more convenient and more precise to equate dose with body weight, height or body surface area. This does not seem to hold true for anticholinergic drugs. A particular dose for an age range works better:

SCOPOLAMINE

I.M. Dose	Age Range
0.1 mg.	Birth to 1 year
0.2 mg.	1 year to 6 years
0.3 mg.	6 years to 10 years
0.4 mg.	10 years to 14 years

4. If the I.V. route is available and easily obtained, we
    give half to two thirds of the above dose and repeat
    as needed—presence or increase of secretions being
    used as the criterion. Our particular choice for in-
    fants and children is *scopolamine* because of the ad-
    vantages mentioned. *Overdosage* in children is quite
    frequent with these drugs, and is often manifested
    by hallucinations, tachycardia, marked flushing, and
    a rise in temperature of as much as 2 to 3 degrees
    Fahrenheit. The *therapeutic* safety range is great,
    however, and even if signs of toxicity should mani-
    fest, these are easily handled with sedation and ad-
    ministration of fluids.

B. NARCOTIC ANALGESICS

1. The use of these drugs in the emergency patient is
    hardly ever necessary unless the patient is in *severe
    pain* and some definitive procedure which will cor-
    rect or remedy the source of pain is contemplated
    immediately. Aside from relieving the pain, a state
    of pharmacologic prefrontal lobotomy also exists
    and the patient is relieved of all fear and worry.
    Some *disadvantages* of this group of drugs are
    respiratory center and cardiovascular depression.
    Advantages would be that the narcotic analgesic ef-
    fects can be reversed by the antagonists and for a
    general anesthetic, the analgesic may continue to
    be used as part of the anesthesia.
2. *Dosage and choice of drug.*—The more commonly
    used narcotic analgesics such as morphine and
    meperidine (Demerol) are easily available in most
    emergency services. The calming effect of narcotics
    in the newborn to 1-year group is rarely needed and
    the respiratory depression which is quite unpredic-
    table in this age group negates the value of the seda-
    tive effect.

    For *meperidine,* the dosage schedules we use are
    as follows:

Dose	Age Range
10 mg.	1 year to 2 years
25 mg.	3 years to 7 years
35-40 mg.	7 years to 9 years
50 mg.	Up to 12 years

A big hulking 12-year-old will easily tolerate up to 75.0 to 100.0 mg. without any difficulty. Respiratory depression is minimal, although hypotension may persist, particularly if sudden postural changes are made.

3. *Morphine* is *10 times* as potent as meperidine, and dosages may be computed on the basis of 1/10 of the meperidine dosages. There are other newer analgesics which are more potent than the two mentioned, but their potency precludes their use for premedication. Since calming effects and analgesia are needed rapidly in the emergency patient, the best route of administration is I.V. if available, otherwise intramuscular.

C. HYPNOTICS AND SEDATIVES

1. We find very little use for these in the emergency pediatric patient. They may be of value in the highly agitated patient. If the patient is in pain, a disturbed type of sleep may prevail and it is not uncommon to find thrashing and screaming. Some amnesia is afforded by the barbiturate and the patient does not remember the disturbance he created. In this situation, a combination of the barbiturate with a narcotic analgesic in small doses to avoid respiratory depression may be of some value.

2. *Choice of Drug and Dosage.* – The short acting oxybarbiturates like secobarbital (Seconal) and pentobarbital (Nembutal) are recommended. Onset and duration of action of the two drugs given parenterally are about equal. We give 25.0 mg., I.M., for

children up to 3 years, 50.0 mg. from 3-8 years, and 75.0 mg. from 8-12 years.

3. They are given I.V. or I.M. The brief and profound respiratory depression observed with I.V. administration of thiobarbiturates, e.g., pentothal is not seen with the oxybarbiturates. In our experience, pentothal works best in combination with scopolamine. The sedative and amnesic effects of this anticholinergic drug is reinforced by the short acting oxybarbiturates.

III. REGIONAL ANESTHESIA

Since this is not meant to be a review of anesthetic procedures, it must be eclectic and pragmatic but not thorough. From the standpoint of the psyche, many children are not able to cope with the thought of suffering pain from a needle no matter how fine or small. On the other hand, there are undoubtedly many children who have had to undergo minor suturing of cuts with infiltration block anesthesia sedated by nothing more than the sympathetic, soothing and hypnotic *voice* of the surgeon.

A. LOCAL INFILTRATION BLOCK WITH OR WITHOUT SEDATION

1. For superficial cuts which necessitate approximation and debridement, this form of anesthesia is the most practical and readily available to the surgeon. The approach is either from within the wound injecting the local anesthetic centrifugally into the tissues or outside the wound infiltrating just lateral to the lips of the wound. The decision to infiltrate with the local from without or within *depends to a great extent* upon factors such as relative cleanliness of the wound and the degree and amount of macerated tissue.

2. Sedation here is of great value. Meperidine or morphine (see dose under premedication) with a mild tranquilizing drug particularly for meperidine will result in a more cooperative and calm patient. The

tranquilizer will diminish the occasional CNS stimulating action of the local anesthetic and the dizziness frequently experienced with meperidine. It will also tend to antagonize any tendency to nausea and vomiting.

3. **Drug of choice.**
   a. Since the anesthetic procedure is a volume block, and peripheral nerves (fibers) are unmyelinated or poorly myelinated, a 0.5% concentration of *procaine hydrochloride* which is the least toxic of the local anesthetics and very quickly metabolized might be the drug of choice.
   b. However, it is quite short-acting, and if a longer procedure is anticipated, 0.5% *Xylocaine* (Lidocaine) solution is recommended. Xylocaine diffuses thru tissues and tissue planes very quickly and a small amount of adrenaline (1:200,000) might be needed to retain the drug longer in the operative site.
   c. *Mepivacaine,* 0.5% does not diffuse as rapidly as Xylocaine and might be more useful for longer procedures.
   d. For *sedation,* our choice is *meperidine,* and promethazine (Phenergan) for the tranquilizer. The *dose* for *promethazine* would be *0.5 mg. per pound body weight* up to a maximum of 50.0 mg. Aside from the tranquilizing, antinauseant and sedative-augmenting effects, promethazine is also an excellent antihistaminic and able to mitigate some of the allergic reactions procaine or the others might provoke.

B. REGIONAL BLOCKS

Two regional anesthesia procedures may be of value in the child for the upper extremity: *the axillary nerve block* and *I.V. Xylocaine block* (see Chap. 5.)

1. *Axillary block.*—For the upper extremity, this block is preferable to the brachial plexus block as it obviates some complications such as pneumothorax. The procedure has been done quite extensively in

children and with mild sedation or some degree of tranquilization, it may be the ideal anesthetic technique for brief surgical procedures from the mid-arm down to the fingers.

a. Anatomically, the axillary nerves are very superficial and readily accessible at the apex of the axilla immediately under the shelf of the pectoralis major muscle. If the arm is extended at right angles from the body, supinated and flexed at the elbow, the *axillary artery* which would be the major guide to the nerves may be seen to pulsate just beneath the skin at the above described site. If not discernible, its pulse beat can be felt when pushed against the *humerus,* which serves as the other major landmark for this block.

b. Since the artery at this point lies in a hollow formed by the four major nerves of the upper extremity, i.e., the median, ulnar, musculocutaneous and radial, staying close to the artery with the block needle even to the point of puncturing it occasionally increases success of the block tremendously. The other factor which will enhance success of block is elicitation of *paresthesias* to the hand (median and ulnar nerves), and to the wrist and forearm (radial and musculocutaneous).

c. Procedure. A 1/4-inch rubber tube tourniquet is placed around the upper arm just distal to the shelf formed by the pectoralis major muscle and tightened enough to compress the artery slightly. The axillary artery is palpated against the humerus with the fore and middle fingers close to the apex of the axilla. A 5/8-inch, 25-gauge needle attached to a 10-ml. syringe containing procaine 2%, or lidocaine, or mepivacaine 1-1.5% is inserted thru a skin wheal between a gap formed by the middle finger and the forefinger, both on the artery, the forefinger proximally and the middle finger distally. In this manner, contact with the artery is maintained despite the obliterative bulk interposed by the injected local anesthetic.

Paresthesias are elicited by probing with the needle, and 3-5 ml. of solution injected every time a paresthesia is provoked. The direction of the needle should always be *perpendicular* to the humerus, but probing should be done close to the artery above, below, and behind the artery for the *radial nerve*. This is always the hardest paresthesia to elicit and can be frustrating in many instances since the hand and the arm may be paralyzed, but some sensation remains around the wrist, the anatomic snuffbox and the dorsal aspect of the hand, thumb, index, middle, and ring fingers.

d. Ten to 20 ml. of local anesthetic solution is sufficient for the child. The tourniquet is *left on* for a period of 5-10 minutes after injection to direct the drug cephalad toward the brachial plexus. This, too, improves effectiveness of the block. Some groups maintain that probing the nerves for paresthesias is not necessary. Our experience shows such probing to greatly increase success in axillary blocks. A block failure always develops an attitude of cynicism toward these procedures on the part of the patient and surgeon.

2. *Intravenous regional anesthesia with lidocaine.* – First performed historically with procaine by Von Bier, this procedure is probably one of the simplest and most effective anesthetic procedures for the arm and hand up to midarm. Availability of a vein on the dorsum of the hand makes the technique more effective especially if the contemplated procedure is on the hand.

a. A 20- or 18-gauge plastic I.V. catheter is inserted into a dorsal hand vein and taped well to the skin. We prefer to attach it to a regular I.V. drip bottle (250-ml. vol.) of physiologic saline (N.S.S.)

or 5% dextrose in water. The injection site on the I.V. tubing, the closest to the needle, is used to introduce the local anesthetic.

b. The I.V. drip is turned off and an Esmarch bandage employed to milk the venous blood proximally. A double-cuffed tourniquet is placed high on the upper arm just below the deltoid muscle and after the upper extremity has been emptied of blood by the Esmarch bandage, the cephalad cuff (proximal) is inflated to 250 mm. Hg pressure. The lidocaine solution, 0.5%, is injected through an injection site on the I.V. tubing as close to the needle as possible. The amount of drug varies from 15 to 30 ml. of the 0.5% solution. Some groups would instill a total dose of 1.5 mg. per pound body weight. Two mg./lb. weight would be closer to the average dose. After instillation of the local anesthetic, the I.V. needle is removed and bleeding at the site stopped by local pressure. After a wait of about 5 or 10 minutes, the distal cuff is inflated, and the cephalad cuff deflated. The distal cuff then would be exerting pressure over an anesthetized area, and diminish the discomfort of feeling excessive pressure on the upper arm under the cuff.

c. After 30 minutes, the cuff may be deflated without fear of flooding the systemic circulation with the local anesthetic. At the end of this period and beyond, it may be assumed that most of the local anesthetic molecules have been absorbed into the lipid tissues, and will be released slowly to be metabolized by the liver.

d. This procedure may be used on the lower extremity with the double-cuffed tourniquet. Because of the greater bulk of tissue to be compressed, a greater pressure of about 500 mm. Hg might be necessary. A vein on the dorsum of the foot just like on the hand would assure sufficient anesthesia of the foot and toes. The use of the Esmarch bandage to milk the extremity of blood is not obligatory. This may be accomplished by holding up the extremity for about 5 minutes to achieve the same objective though perhaps not as efficiently. We have had very little experience in I.V. regional anesthesia of the lower extremity, but it does not seem to be a formidable procedure. Considering the bulk of the lower extremity as compared to the upper extremity, a volume of 25-40 ml. of a 0.5% solution of local anesthetic might be needed to achieve the same degree of anesthesia as in the upper extremity.

IV. ABDOMEN AND LOWER EXTREMITIES

A. *Epidural anesthesia* should certainly be considered. The epidural space is a potential space between the dura and the ligamentum flavum. Location of this space is somewhat difficult. A special spinal needle with a rounded end, preferably a Touhy, and with a sharp stylet extending beyond the rounded end is helpful.
   1. The needle is introduced thru the second or third lumbar space until the interspinous ligament is encountered. The stylet is removed and a 2-ml. glass syringe containing a milliliter of air is attached to the hub of the needle. The piston of the syringe should be lubricated well with either local anesthetic or NSS. Slight pressure on the piston will show marked resistance to injection so the piston "bounces" back. The needle is slowly and cautiously advanced continuously repeating the air-injection technique. As soon as the epidural space is entered, resistance to injection is suddenly lost and the air is easily injected into the epidural space.
   2. Local anesthetic such as lidocaine 1% or procaine 2% is instilled. There should be no resistance to injection. The amount of anesthetic will vary from 10 to 20 ml. depending on the age and weight. The procedure works best in the 5-12-year age group. If

the dura is inadvertently entered, spinal fluid will usually gush out. A spinal anesthetic should then be considered.

B. *Spinal.* – The youngest patient we have ever given a spinal anesthetic to was 4-5 years old. The preferred drug is tetracaine, which comes as niphanoid crystals or 1% solution. The dose used never exceeded 5 mg. in a hyperbaric solution with dextrose 10%. The duration of anesthesia is from 60 to 90 minutes. Hypotension may be prevented by injecting 5-10 mg. ephedrine I.M.

V. GENERAL ANESTHESIA (GENERAL CONSIDERATIONS)

If trauma to a child's pysche is imminent, then a general anesthetic is much better than regional anesthesia. Induction should be quick and pleasant, maintenance relatively problem-free and recovery untroubled. There will be no attempt to dwell upon the merits and deficiencies of any agent or technique; instead, we will emphasize agents and techniques that are pragmatically utilizable in the Emergency Service. Because of the ever present threat of vomiting and aspiration, *intubation* may be mandatory and availability of *very good suction* a necessity. *Monitoring devices* must be available and used.

A. DRUGS OR COMBINATION OF DRUGS

1. There are three drugs or groups of drugs which satisfy the brief but mandatory requirements for general anesthetics that may be employed for the emergency pediatric patient. These drugs are: (1) ketamine, (2) narcotic analgesics and nitrous oxide and (3) nitrous oxide and halothane.

2. *Ketamine HCl.* – This drug may well be one of the outstanding discoveries of anesthesia. Only time and usage, however, will judge eventually whether this drug has found a proper niche in the armamentarium or be relegated to obscurity. We are inclined to believe at the moment that it is almost ideal for

the brief surgical procedure, anything lasting from 1 minute to 1 hour at the maximum. Beyond this time limit, the patient will tend to sleep longer, ambulation is delayed and the value to the patient somehow diminished. I.V. or I.M. induction is very rapid—the patient going to sleep within 30 seconds after I.V. injection, and within 3 minutes on the average after I.M. injection. It provides *profound general anesthesia* for a brief period of time, 10-15 minutes for an I.V. dose and around 30-45 minutes for the I.M. dose.

a. The effect on autonomic functions is minimal. Respiration may be momentarily depressed but not to the point of provoking marked changes in the blood gas picture; Pco_2, Po_2, and pH remain within normal limits. The blood pressure rises and the pulse rate may increase after induction but usually comes back to normal within 10-15 minutes. We have not noted any arrhythmias, but then the briefness of the procedures did not warrant application of a monitor. Arrhythmias, bradycardias, and hypotension have been observed.

b. One advantage or disadvantage of this drug is maintenance of laryngeal and pharyngeal reflexes. Although presence of pharyngeal reflexes maintains patency of the oropharyngeal airway and enables the patient to swallow secretions or even vomitus or regurgitated material, active *laryngeal* reflexes may be stimulated to cause varying degrees of *laryngospasm* which can give rise to severe *hypoxia* and even cardiac arrest.

c. Nausea and vomiting in postanesthesia has been minimized but it does occur. One of the most unpleasant aftermaths of ketamine, though observed *mostly in adults* is the occurrence of *hallucinations,* sometimes very vivid, disturbing, and unpleasant. It may be obviated by the administration of small doses of pentothal (25-50 mg.) or tranquilizers.

    d.   The I.V. *dose* is 1-2 mg./lb. body wt., which
should provide general anesthesia for around 15
minutes. If another 15 minutes of anesthesia
time is contemplated, a similar amount is given.
There is a cumulative effect so that in the third
and fourth 15-minute periods, only *half* the dose
should be given. The average I.M. dose is 5
mg./lb. body weight. Here, since absorption is
slower, the onset is slower, but the state of
anesthesia is maintained longer, about 30-45
minutes. Additional dosage for longer anesthesia,
e.g., the next 30-minute period should be *no*
greater than *half* the initial dose.

    e.   Ketamine has been employed successfully and
to great advantage in such diverse procedures as
operations in the eye, ear, nose, and mouth
areas, orthopedic procedures, debridement and
skin grafts, pneumoencephalograms, ventriculo-
grams, minor surgery of the anus and rectum,
circumcision and minor gynecologic operations.

3. *Narcotic analgesics and nitrous oxide.* – The main
disadvantage of narcotic analgesics is respiratory
depression. This can be mitigated by augmenting
respiration by means of an anesthesia machine and
administration of nitrous oxide with the oxygen at
a ratio of 50:50 which reduces the amount of narcotic analgesic needed. For induction of anesthesia,
the narcotic analgesic is a poor agent. A huge dose
is needed to bring about the sleep state; such a dose
will frequently cause cardiovascular depression. Introduction of an inducing agent such as thiopental
given intravenously or rectally complicates the
anesthesia greatly as its hypnotic effects are not as
readily reversible compared to reversibility of the
narcotic analgesic effects with a narcotic antagonist.

    a.   The analgetic drug of choice for maintenance
would be *meperidine.* The initial dose is 25-50
mg. I.V. followed by increments of 5-10 mg. to
maintain a minimal effective concentration in
the blood stream monitored by reactions of the

patient to surgical stimuli. Addition of a tranquilizing drug such as Phenergan will potentiate the narcotic effect but might also prolong the action. It is assumed that *endotracheal intubation* is used as vomiting and aspiration are always a possibility and a hazard.

b. Recently, a combination of a very potent narcotic and a long acting tranquilizer had become quite popular. This combination is Innovar. It is composed of a short acting, very potent narcotic, *sublimaze,* which is 150-200 times as potent as morphine, and *droperidol,* a tranquilizer. Expertise and experience are needed in the use of this drug combination.

4. *Nitrous-halothane anesthesia.* — For induction and maintenance, this gas-vapor combination satisfies the criteria initially noted. Both provide pleasant and rapid induction. Maintenance for short procedures has minimal problems particularly if emphasis is laid on using nitrous oxides as the primary agent and halothane as a supplement. The possibility of provoking *halothane hepatitis* has become a kind of millstone that has tended to drag this technique down, but reports of hepatitis in children from halothane have been few and far between. *Intubation* is indicated.

B. METHODS OF INHALATION ANESTHESIA

1. *Open or semiopen technique.*
   a. The *open technique,* which is best exemplified by an Ayre's T-piece, is nothing more than a hollow tube with a side arm. Ideally, the side arm should equal the tidal volume of the patient. Increasing the volume of the side arm will bring about re-breathing and thus tachypnea from the CO_2. Jackson Rees has modified the system by adding an open-tailed breathing bag attached to a length of corrugated tubing to the side arm. Capability of controlling respiration

is then possible. In this technique, gas flow from the anesthesia machine should be at least twice the minute volume to diminish or eliminate re-breathing.

   b. The *semiopen* technique implies the use of a *unidirectional* valve interposed between the patient and a breathing bag and the source of gas. There are several types available, e.g., the Digby-Leigh valve, the Stephen-Slater valve, the Fink valve, and Ruben valve, etc. The Fink and the Ruben valves enable the operator to assist or control respiration without having to occlude the exhalation port on compressing the breathing bag.

2. *Semiclosed and closed techniques.*

   a. The current most accepted connotation of the term *semiclosed* in inhalation anesthesia technique is high gas flow in a circle system (with soda lime interposed) and excess gas vented to the atmosphere through a pop-off valve. In the utilization of a gas-oxygen-vapor mixture, e.g., nitrous oxide-oxygen-halothane, the semiclosed technique is commonly employed.

   b. The *closed* circle, which requires the presence of soda lime for CO_2 absorption in the system and a low flow of gases, does not work well with gas-oxygen-vapor mixture. The debate has been whether adult-size circle units may be used in infants and children or should special children units (which are available) be used exclusively. Studies show that adult units may be used in infants and children particularly if respiration is assisted or controlled.

C. SPECIAL PROCEDURES AND EQUIPMENT

1. *Endotracheal intubation.* – Because of the frequency of vomiting and aspiration in emergency patients who are given general anesthesia, it is a rule that all such patients be intubated. The question that always arises is--should these patients be intubated *awake* or

after induction as is done routinely? An awake patient of course is able to avoid aspiration, should he vomit. Such a procedure may only be done with difficulty in the child. It is not too difficult in the 0-1 year group. Above this age, it gets decidedly more so, unless the child might be debilitated, in which case, he is less prone to fight against the procedure.

a. It is possible to sedate the child with a *narcotic analgesic* at the temporary risk of depressing his respiration and cardiovascular state. If the intubation is accomplished quickly, the untoward actions of the narcotic analgesic may be immediately reversed with an antagonist such as levallorphan (Lorfan). Optimal effects of the narcotic and the antagonist are best given *intravenously*.

b. If an awake intubation is not possible, a *"crash induction"* should be done. A quick but not too rapid injection of *pentothal sodium—1.0 mg./lb. body wt.* followed by *succinylcholine, also 1.0 mg./lb. body wt. but not to exceed 60 mg.* is used for induction. Intubation is then accomplished as rapidly as possible after the relaxant has become effective.

c. Certain maneuvers may be performed to prevent stomach content regurgitation, e.g., placing the patient in the Fowler position, compression of the cricoid cartilage against the esophageal sphincter, which maneuver also facilitates intubation.

   Good suction must be available. If the patient can tolerate oxygen by mask before induction for 7-10 minutes, manual inflation of the lungs with the anesthesia bag will not be necessary after the succinylcholine.

d. Equipment.—A laryngoscope is necessary for this procedure. An infant, child, and a medium adult blade (for bigger children) should be available. As to the type of blade, we have no

particular preference, although we have found
the Miller blade to be quite versatile and adapta-
ble to many situations.

1) The *endotracheal tube* with a cuff that may
   be inflated to occlude the space around the
   tube in the trachea is used. However, the
   presence of a cuff tends to encroach upon
   the diameter of the tube, and in the child's
   small trachea, a very small decrease in the
   diameter can represent a markedly disproportionate decrease in the airway area since
   laminar airflow according to Poiseuille's law
   is directly proportional to the fourth power
   of the radius. Turbulent flow makes this
   worse.

2) The endotracheal tube in the child has certain *disadvantages*. It is frequent to find
   laryngeal and tracheal mucosal edema in
   children below the age of 10 after endotracheal intubation. The edema can cause
   so much obstruction, particularly at the region of the cricoid where the trachea is nar-
   rowest, as to necessitate (in some instances)
   a tracheostomy. Most of the time, conservative treatment, including oxygen, high humidity, epinephrine vapor inhalation or
   spray to the area may allow the condition to
   subside. Our experience has shown that the
   chances of provoking laryngeal and tracheal
   edema increases with the *length of time* the
   tube stays in the trachea. In brief procedures, therefore, chances of edema developing are almost minimal.

e. *Suction.*—Most general anesthetics stimulate the
   production of secretions in the oropharyngeal
   area and trachea. This may be minimized by injection of anticholinergics such as atropine and
   scopolamine. Fear, which seems to stimulate
   cholinergic responses apparently augments the
   production of secretions. In the emergency

patient, both the general anesthetic and fear combine to provoke nausea and vomiting. Usual presence of stomach contents in these patients makes the immediate availability of *excellent suction imperative.* Stiff, preferably metal suction tips such as used in tonsillectomies are better than the soft plastic catheters.

f. *Monitoring.* – The simplest monitor, quite efficient, is the stethoscope. Equally simple is the strength and rate of the pulse, and watching the character and rate of respiration. In the child and infant, the strength of the heart sound is crudely proportional to the effective blood pressure. *Breath sounds,* character or absence (apnea due to obstruction, breath-holding, or depression of respiratory center), may also be monitored at the same time through the same stethoscope.

1) The stethoscope may be taped to the precordial area, or the child made to lie on it and located opposite to but somewhat medial to the precordial area in the back. An esophageal stethoscope is more efficient than a chest stethoscope. A recently devised esophageal stethoscope also includes an ECG electrode.

2) A blood pressure cuff (child's and infant sizes) and a sphygmomanometer are also good monitors but quite cumbersome for the short procedure and not efficient in the infant.

3) A finger or toe plethysmograph (pulse sensor) and an electrocardiograph, both displayed on an oscilloscope, give an excellent assessment of cardiovascular status particularly in the infant. A display of good pulse height, regular in rate from the plethysmograph indicates good peripheral blood flow.

4) Early shock causes peripheral vasoconstriction and the pulse wave diminishes and

almost disappears even if what seems to be a good blood pressure is discernible; peripheral blood flow and flow to organs may be poor.

5) The ECG is also a good index of cardiac status, and immediate recognition of arrhythmias enables the anesthesiologist or monitoring personnel to correct quickly the conditions that may be causing them.

6) The ultimate in monitoring would be *computerized interpretation* of parametric data obtained from an indwelling arterial catheter such as blood pressure, pulse pressure, pulse rate, cardiac output, peripheral resistance, ventricular work, etc.

7) An indwelling central venous catheter for status of the right heart, respiratory rate, and venous return is helpful. A bonus from the arterial catheter would be ability to determine blood gases—pH, Pco_2, Po_2, buffer base or base excess. The possibility of determining cations and anions in blood from either the artery or the CVP also becomes quite simple, particularly if the equipment is available.

2. *Recovery room.*—If any form of anesthesia is administered in the Emergency Service, a postanesthesia room for the patient is mandatory. Trained nurses, technicians, and aides who are able to recognize sudden and acute changes in vital functions should observe the patient. *Monitoring* equipment should be available, and so should all drugs and equipment needed for resuscitation. The ratio of the number of recovery room beds to each Emergency Service operating area will depend somewhat on the volume of patients handled. A minimum of 4 PAR beds to each operating area may be sufficient.

CHAPTER 23

Otolaryngologic Emergencies

FRANCIS L. LEDERER, M.D.,* LOUIS T. TENTA, M.D., *and* M. EUGENE TARDY, JR., M.D.

I. FOREIGN BODY IN AIR AND FOOD PASSAGES

A. PROCEDURE

Evaluate the airway.

B. HISTORY

Try to identify the object, time of ingestion or aspiration, previous attempts at removal or home treatment, prior air and food-passage problems or disorders, emotional status of patient or other serious illnesses. The finding of certain foreign bodies is common in a particular age group: safety pin, coin or peanut in a child; dentures, food boli and bones in adults. Fishbones are most often found in the faucial tonsil or the base of the tongue in the lingual tonsil. Safety pins, coins and dentures often lodge in the cricopharyngeal area; and smaller objects, such as tacks and peanuts, are frequently found in the trachea or bronchi. The foreign bodies may be multiple. Be aware that some previously unrecognized problem, such as an esophageal stricture or a psychotic state, may exist. Wherever possible, acquire a duplicate of the foreign body or the object from which the foreign body was removed.

C. SYMPTOMS AND SIGNS

The symptoms are: agitation, drooling, site pain, referred pains, odynophagia (pain on swallowing), stridor,

---

*Deceased.

respiratory distress, cough, hoarseness, dysphagia, hematemesis and possibly cyanosis. Occasionally only a history of a possible foreign body ingestion or aspiration is elicited and the patient may otherwise be symptomless. In these instances, meticulous investigation and surveillance are indicated.

D. PHYSICAL EXAMINATION

Examine the mouth, pharynx, larynx and neck tissues. Signs of segmental obstruction, an audible thud and/or localized wheezing may be evident on auscultation of the chest. Recognize the complications of a foreign body in a solid or hollow viscus, namely, obstruction, perforation and/or hemorrhage.

E. X-RAY

Roentgenograms may include all anatomic regions from the nasopharynx to the pelvic floor in anteroposterior and lateral views. The arms should be held up and back out of the airway and esophageal shadows. Inspiratory and expiratory x-ray films of the chest in frontal and lateral projections are indicated in aspirated nonopaque foreign bodies. They aid in the recognition of an endobronchial check-valve system which may be a consequence of the foreign body. Characteristic areas of hyper- and/or hypoventilation of the lungs with mediastinal shifts may be demonstrated. *Radiographic contrast media* are to be avoided in the initial appraisal. Frontal and lateral projections of the neck for soft tissue detail are of decided value. **Have otolaryngologic physician review all cases.**

Avoid the use of emetic agents. Do not compound the foreign body problem by adding other foreign bodies (asking patient to eat bread, swallow water, etc.).

II. FOREIGN BODIES IN THE NOSE OR EAR CANAL

Ascertain, if possible, the type of foreign body and whether previous attempts at removal were made. Any object small enough to pass into the nostril or external ear openings may be found lodged in these areas. Such objects are frequently wedged in, owing to unskilled attempts at removal. The problem in a child may be complicated by his reluctance or inability to cooperate.

A. SIGNS AND SYMPTOMS

1. *Nose.* – Pain, sneezing or unilateral nasal obstruction may be late, rather than early, complaints. Later, some bleeding, accompanied by fetor and foul discharge, are significant findings.
2. *Ear.* – Late signs in the ear may resemble external otitis or chronic ofitis media.
3. *Procedure.* – History and examination, together, suggest the diagnosis. Unskilled attempts at removal of foreign bodies are to be avoided. Essential necessary features are: (1) a cooperative patient (which may imply the use of general anesthesia), (2) proper illumination of the cavity and (3) suitable instruments.

III. INGESTION OF CAUSTICS

This does not include all poisons—only the contact-necrotizing agents. Acids and alkalis used in household cleaning are the most common offenders: lye, ammonia, potassium permanganate, sulfuric acid, etc.

A. HISTORY

Ascertain time, quantity and nature of material ingested. The reason for ingestion and the past emotional behavioral pattern of the patient are important. Careful notations are important because there are often medicolegal implications.

B. PHYSICAL EXAMINATION

Examination of the oral cavity, pharynx and larynx may reveal marked reddening of the mucosa, denuded areas and a coagulum or ulceration, depending on the quantity and quality of caustic agent and the duration of its local action. General status, vital signs and vital organ functions are to be assessed. Airway evaluation is essential, and tracheotomy may be required.

C. LABORATORY STUDIES

These should include: appropriate blood and urine studies and frontal and lateral chest x-ray films and lateral neck x-ray films for soft tissue detail.

D. TREATMENT

Give specific antidote if within 45 minutes of ingestion. Neutralize acid with sodium bicarbonate solution and, for alkalis, use half-strength vinegar. Cooking oils (olive oil in milk) in sips may comfort the patient. Analgesics may be required. Avoid the use of emetic agents. Defer passage of Levine, Ewald or other nasogastric tubes in corrosive esophagitis. If burns are suggested by history and physical examination, the patient should be admitted to the hospital. The extent of Emergency Room therapy depends on the degree of injury. The sites of predilection for chemical burns of the food passage are those areas where there is a physiologic pause or hesitation in deglutition, namely, the lip and the buccal sulcus, palate, tongue, mesopharynx and hypopharynx, the aortic arch and left mainstem bronchus encroachment on the esophagus, the cardia of the esophagus and the stomach. Emotionally disturbed patients require special precautions so as to avoid further attempts at self-destruction. Psychiatric consultation in these patients is indicated.

IV. EMERGENCY TRACHEOTOMY

A. INDICATIONS

Airway obstructions above the suprasternal notch which are not amenable to more specific immediate therapy necessitate tracheotomy. Inspiratory stridor, the use of accessory muscles of respiration, varying degrees of cyanosis, restlessness and pulse elevation are signs of upper respiratory tract obstruction. Narcotics and depressants are to be avoided in instances of respiratory obstruction and respiratory depression.

B. ETIOLOGY

Bilateral choanal atresia in the newborn and other congenital anomalies and tumors, trauma and inflammation of the pharynx, larynx and trachea cause serious airway problems. Foreign bodies should also be considered as well as bilateral inferior laryngeal nerve obstruction.

C. PHYSICAL EXAMINATION

Check patency of nasal passages, using tuft of cotton or mirror to reveal air current at the nostrils or by passage of a no. 10 rubber catheter. Examine the pharynx and larynx with laryngeal mirror whenever possible. A direct laryngeal spatula (Flagg) may be useful. Are there supraclavicular and/or intercostal or sternal retractions? Check voice quality, presence of stridor, wheeze and cry. Review chest findings, cardiac status, and effect of position changes.

D. PROCEDURE

Except in the presence of severe edema, tumor or laryngeal foreign body, the *immediate* insertion of an *oral endotracheal tube* may be lifesaving and serve as a helpful guide during tracheotomy, particularly in children. The trachea usually will tolerate an intubation tube approximately the diameter of the patient's little finger. A *standardized tray of instruments* and supplies for tracheotomy should be available at all times.

E. STEPS OF ORDERLY TRACHEOTOMY

1. Control patient's movements by body wrap if

necessary and have head and neck extended and maintained in position.

2. Adequate lighting is essential.

3. Have a tracheotomy set present, and be familiar with the instruments.

4. Assistance is needed.

5. Suction should be available and tested.

6. Prepare skin if time permits.

7. Infiltrate midline neck tissues with a local anesthetic agent. Because of the existing hypercarbia, catecholamines are to be employed with caution.

8. Incise in the midline from the cricoid cartilage (which is the first ring below the thyroid cartilage and the only complete ring of the trachea) to the suprasternal notch.

9. Carry the incision down to the strap muscles, bluntly separating them. Remain in the midline.

10. Delineate the cricoid cartilage. It is a useful guide. Its integrity must be preserved.

11. Mobilize the thyroid isthmus, control with clamps and transect. This maneuver is necessary only if the isthmus covers the area of the second and third tracheal rings.

12. Obtain hemostasis and transfix the transected thyroid isthmus. Absorbable suture material is preferred. This can be postponed so that it follows steps 15 and 16.

13. Anesthetize the trachea by intraluminal injection of a suitable topical anesthetic with a protected needle. Be certain that the needle is in the trachea by aspirating air prior to instillation. Do not penetrate the common party wall between the trachea and esophagus.

14. Fix and advance trachea with tracheal hook secured in the cricoid cartilage.

15. Make a transverse incision, usually between the second and third tracheal rings. Grasp the rings with suitable forceps and remove a *small semilunar* portion of the anterior wall cartilage in adults. Do not transect the trachea. Protect your eyes from

material that may be coughed out of the patient's trachea. In infants and young children, avoid removal of tracheal cartilage by employing a cruciate incision between and through to greater or lesser degrees of two consecutive rings. Preserve the cricoid cartilage! Do not penetrate the common party wall between the trachea and esophagus.

16. Check conformity and compliance of the inner and outer tracheotomy cannulas with one another prior to their insertion. Insert outer tracheotomy tube with obturator. Remove obturator and insert inner cannula. Be certain that the cannulas are in the trachea. Secure tracheotomy tube tape in square knot at back or side of neck.

17. Avoid air tight closure of incision, since subcutaneous emphysema may result when patient coughs.

18. Aspirate secretions and blood from the trachea. Be prepared for the apnea and profound cardiovascular collapse which may be immediate sequelae following the relief of obstruction and restoration of the airway in the hypercarbic, hypoanoxemic patients.

F. CONIOTOMY (Cricothyrotomy)

The emergency tracheotomy provides a rapid means of entering the airway above the level of the cricoid cartilage. A transverse skin incision is made between the *thyroid* cartilage above and *cricoid* cartilage below, exposing the paired cricothyroid muscles beneath, which is the cricothyroid membrane. The membrane is incised and the airway entered and maintained. An orderly tracheotomy then follows.

G. TRACHEOTOMY CARE

1. Use continuous high humidity as a mist.
2. Sterile tracheal aspiration is needed intermittently.
3. Cleanse inner cannula periodically to prevent crusting.
4. The initial tracheotomy tube changing must be done cautiously.

5. Be alert for complications (hemorrhage, pneumothorax, expulsion of tracheotomy tubes, perforation
   of tracheoesophageal party wall, subcutaneous emphysema, etc.).
6. The patient usually adjusts in a period of 3-5 days,
   requiring less humidity and aspiration. Postoperative
   chest x-ray films and blood gas studies are valuable
   parameters and indicators.

V. ACUTE EXTERNAL OTITIS
(Diffuse or Circumscribed)

A. SYMPTOMS

Pain in the ear, especially on chewing or with pressure
on the tragus or a full feeling in the ear with a sense of
hearing loss. Referred pains to head and neck are frequent.

B. OBJECTIVE FINDINGS

Pain on lifting pinna, from pressure on tragus or on
inspection of canal. The meatus and canal vary in the
degree of swelling—to the extent that the drum may not
be visualized. The patient also may have an otitis media.
Secretions may be present.

C. TREATMENT

Gently wipe or aspirate debris from canal which may
be inoculated into a suitable culture media or prepared
for bacteriologic staining. The canal may be so tender
and swollen that it is difficult to rule out a perforation
of the drum head or the presence of a foreign body.
Swelling behind the ear may mimic mastoiditis, and
slight fever may be present, as well as decreased hearing.
Instill Burow's solution, 1:10, 4 or 5 drops 4 times a day
either directly in the ear canal or on a selvage-edge (1/4-
inch) gauze wick which has been inserted gently into the
canal. Very soothing and rapidly acting are the anti-
flammatory, antibiotic, antifungal agents in the form of

otic drops. Systemic antibiotics may be indicated. Analgesics systemically are required in adequate dosage. Re-examine the patient in 3-4 days to a week for toilet of the ear, otoscopy and acoustic function evaluation.

VI. TRAUMATIC PERFORATION OF THE EARDRUM

A. SYMPTOMS

Frequently there is pain and bleeding from the ear, hearing loss, fullness and tinnitus. Vertigo, though possible, is not likely. There may be a history of a slap on the ear, head injury or ear trauma (toothpick, needle, etc.).

B. EVALUATION

In tuning fork study, in an otherwise normally hearing individual, the Weber test will lateralize to the affected ear; usually Rinne's test will be negative (bone conduction dominating air) in the affected ear and positive (air conduction exceeding bone conduction) on the normal side. Observe for the presence of nystagmus and check function of seventh and other cranial nerves.

C. TREATMENT

Keep instruments and medication out of the ear. If absolutely necessary, use a sterile speculum or suction tip to evaluate the drum findings. Avoid contamination of the ear. Secondary infection may cause suppuration. Acute perforations may benefit from immediate otosurgical closure. Use sterile cotton to obturate loosely the ear canal. Give a broad spectrum antibiotic for 5 days. Surveillance and reappraisal otologically and audiologically are indicated as might be other laboratory or radiographic studies.

VII. ACUTE OTITIS MEDIA

A. HISTORY

Frequently associated with an upper respiratory infection, or as a sequela.

B. SYMPTOMS

Otalgia, hearing loss, head pains, full head ("all blocked up" feeling) are the complaints. Note that in a young child this may reflect a serous otitis media even though there is only a slight fever. In the adult a condition characterized by vesicles—myringitis bullosa—may be present.

C. PHYSICAL FINDINGS

Early in the course of the disease, there may be noted only dilated vessels on the eardrum. An injected drum with altered light reflex is observed. The position of the malleus, Shrapnell's membrane, drum rim and light reflex are helpful in evaluating the condition of the middle ear. Decide if the drum is bulging or in a normal, slightly indrawn position. Pulsation or a perforation may be seen. Fever and malaise are common. The Weber test will usually lateralize to the affected ear. Rinne's test is most likely to be negative in the affected ear and positive in the normal ear.

D. TREATMENT

If the patient is quite toxic or if there is severe ear pain, myringotomy may be necessary. A red, bulging eardrum warrants myringotomy and culture and bacteriologic stain analysis of the exudate. Earlier in the course of the disease, progression of symptoms may be aborted by the use of systemic antibiotics, preferably penicillin, and local or systemic nasal decongestants.

E. PROCEDURE OF MYRINGOTOMY

1. Explain the procedure to the patient, since his co-operation is essential.
2. Young patients must be immobilized; sedation or general anesthesia may be required.
3. Cleanse the ear canal.
4. Local or topical anesthesia may be employed but is of limited value.
5. Use a sterile, sharp myringotomy knife. Steady the instrument with your hand on the side of the patient's head. Good light and accurate orientation are essential. Incise the eardrum in its inferior-posterior quadrant. Begin the incision anteriorly and direct it posteriorly, since the drum slopes from medial to lateral as one proceeds posteriorly.
6. Aspirate the fluid return and prepare it for bacteriologic studies. Prescribe systemic antibiotic, nasal decongestant, and anodyne.

F. *Serous* otitis may be relieved by aspiration of the fluid by means of a 20-gauge needle. The chronic draining ear without toxic neurologic manifestations is ordinarily not a medical emergency. However, it may lead to an acute otitis externa or be subject to an acute exacerbation.

VIII. FURUNCLE IN THE NASAL VESTIBULE

A furuncle in the nasal vestibule is potentially dangerous as a possible cause of cavernous sinus thrombosis, just as is any infection above the upper lip. Abstinence from manipulation is the best policy.

A. OBJECTIVE FINDINGS

Classic signs of infection in a hair follicle of the nasal vestibule are tenderness and redness of the lobule of nose.

B. TREATMENT

1. Culture material from exudate, if present.
2. Systemic broad spectrum antibiotic in adequate dosage.
3. Antibiotic ointment applied intranasally.
4. Heat applications to nose every 3 hours.
5. Incise only if fluctuant and focally necrotic—then under most aseptic precautions. Otherwise, be most conservative. Obtain bacteriologic specimen.

IX. EPISTAXIS

Most instances of epistaxis occur from the anterior portion of the nose along the septum. In the young, the cause is usually digital trauma. Epistaxis frequently follows a head cold. To be ruled out are nasal tumors, trauma, foreign body, hypertension or a hematologic disturbance.

A. PROCEDURE

Have all equipment set out on a tray and the procedure planned. Diagnose the site and cause of the bleeding.

1. Have head mirror and adequate light.
2. Have suction apparatus and nasal aspirating tips.
3. Position patient appropriately, usually in a semirecumbent position.
4. Protect yourself and the patient with aprons or gowns.
5. Give the patient a basin into which blood and secretions may be expectorated.
6. Aspirate all clots and debris from the nose.
7. Check pharynx for bleeding posteriorly.
8. Spray the nose with an appropriate topical anesthetic. Catecholamines are to be employed cautiously in the hypertensive patient. If there is a heavy flow of blood, pack the nose quickly with a couple of large cotton pledgets dampened lightly in a suitable topical anesthetic. Lay them over the area of bleeding.

9. When the bleeding point is identified, chemical cautery may be employed by application of silver nitrate or trichloroacetic acid. This will stop most nosebleeds. A hyfrecator (electrocoagulation unit plus suction) may be employed.

10. If the bleeding is stopped, emphasize that the patient should not manipulate the nose or engage in exceptional activity for several days. Be sure that the general medical condition is satisfactory.

11. If the patient is still bleeding after the above procedure, anterior packing of 1-inch lubricated gauze stripping is layered from the floor to the roof of the nose.

12. Attempt repeatedly, with the nose anesthetized, to locate and cauterize a bleeding point prior to resorting to lubricated gauze packing.

13. If the patient is still bleeding or if the examination demonstrates the bleeding to be posterior in the nose, insert a posterior nasopharyngeal pack and pack anteriorly against it through the nose.

B. METHOD OF INSERTION OF A POSTERIOR NASAL PACK

1. Anesthetize the pharynx, soft palate and nose with a small amount of an appropriate topical anesthetic spray. A posterior pack readiness tray is usually present in the Emergency Service. The posterior nasal pack is a snug roll of gauze approximately 1 inch in all its dimensions. Three stout cords are secured to the tampon. Some prefer to fashion a miniature cone out of the gauze, using two sutures, and to draw up the tapered end of the cone into one posterior choana.

2. Lubricate the pack (a broad spectrum antibiotic ointment may be preferred). Insert one no. 12F catheter through the nostril identified as the site of bleeding, retrieve it in the pharynx and bring it out of the mouth with a hemostat. Tie two of the tampon cords to the oral end of the catheter. Withdraw

the catheter through the nose, thereby drawing the cords through the nose and guiding the tampon in the postnasal space. With the direct finger pressure, push the pack firmly against the posterior choana. The cords are then detached from the catheter. The third cord may be cut short and left to dangle in the throat or brought out the mouth and taped loosely to the cheek; it will be used in the subsequent withdrawal of the postnasal pack. Have an aid hold the nasal strings tautly, and firmly pack vaseline gauze into the nose anteriorly against the tampon. Protect the nostril and columella with a soft batten about which are anchored the nasal cords.

3. An alternative method of postnasal tamponade utilizes the insertion of a lubricated no. 18 (no. 12 in children) 30cc. Foley catheter, the projecting tip of which has been cut off, through the anterior nares until it is visible posteriorly at the level of the velum, inflated to 8cc. with saline, withdrawn until it is engaged in the choanae and then inflated to 10-12cc. and anchored. Anterior tamponade follows. The patient with a posterior and anterior pack in place *should be admitted to the hospital.* Prophylactic antibiotic and supportive therapy is warranted.

X. PERITONSILLAR ABSCESS

A. HISTORY

Recurrent sore throats which frequently resolve with one "shot" of penicillin. This sore throat has progressed.

B. SYMPTOMS

Weakness, thirst, chills, fever, odynophagia, ear and neck pains referred from the throat, and trismus are common. Trismus pain, which is characteristic, may prevent the patient from opening his mouth to allow adequate inspection.

C. OBJECTIVE FINDINGS

The patient is toxic and febrile; also noted: thick speech, drooling, trismus, contralateral displacement of the edematous uvula and a tonsil that is beefy red and advancing to the midline. There is a fullness at the juncture of the soft palate and lateral margin of the palatine tonsil. Cervical adenopathy frequently is present.

D. TREATMENT: INCISION AND DRAINAGE

1. Explain the procedure to the patient.
2. *Instruments:* No. 11 or 15 scalpel blade and handle, tonsil suction tip, metal tongue depressor, topical anesthetic spray, 6- or 8-inch curved hemostat, emesis basin and culture tube.
3. Have the patient properly positioned, somewhat recumbent. Spray the tonsil area lightly with the topical anesthetic. This same agent applied to the posterior end of the middle turbinate on the involved side may aid in lessening trismus. Aspiration of the peritonsillar space prior to incision and drainage may relieve some of the trismus, provide suitable bacteriologic material and aid in excluding the possibility of incising into a great vessel. Incise the mucosa with long-handled bistoury knife at the upper outer pole of the tonsil, where it meets the soft palate. Have the patient's head tilted somewhat forward over emesis basin and spread incision transversely in the peritonsillar space with a hemostat. Obtain culture; facilitate this by use of capillary suction. Do *not* squeeze out pus.
4. Prescribe appropriate antibiotics and pain medications.

XI. ACUTE SINUSITIS

A. MAXILLARY SINUSITIS

1. *History.* —Onset after an upper respiratory infection, facial trauma or a tooth extraction.

2. *Symptoms.* – Nasal blockage, pain over the involved sinus, fever, chills, malaise, dry throat and vague orbital discomfort.

3. *Objective findings.* – Tenderness, swelling, warmth and redness over the involved sinus. Intranasal examination may reveal injected swollen turbinates and mucous membranes. Pus is seldom seen in the very acute stage. The teeth may be sensitive to percussion. Check for dental focus of infection, especially if toothache is an early symptom. Intranasal anatomic variations, such as a markedly deviated nasal septum, may be a causal factor, in that normal ventilation is impaired.

4. *Treatment.* – The principle to be applied is to provide for better nasal and sinus ventilation and drainage. Culture of secretions is desirable. Prescribe the following: a systemic or local nasal decongestant, an appropriate antibiotic, high fluid intake, humidification of the environment, analgesics and bed rest. Close observation is needed, a drainage-irrigation procedure possibly may be required in the subacute stage.

B. *Frontal sinusitis* will have findings localized over the forehead. Therapy is the same.

C. *Acute ethmoiditis* has similar findings. Since the ethmoids line the medial wall of the orbit, orbital swelling, especially in children, may ensue. Therapy is the same.

XII. VERTIGO

Vertigo may present as an acute emergency, with the story that the patient has not been able to move or even be undressed because each movement brings on nausea and vomiting. Among some of the causes of vertigo are: head trauma (concussion and/or temporal bone fracture), intracranial or extracranial vascular disorders affecting the internal auditory artery or its cochlear or vestibular branches, labyrinthitis secondary to suppurative middle ear disease, or possibly of viral cause, toxic origin (such as from drugs) and endolymphatic hydrops.

Tinnitus and varying degrees of hearing loss may be associated. The presence of a spontaneous nystagmus, especially on moving the head, is pathognomonic. If the eyes are open, they often rotate toward the affected side—viz., in the position in which the spontaneous nystagmus and dizziness are decreased. Under the circumstances mentioned, in which the slightest movement of the head leads to violent symptoms, the history looms importantly and complements the physical findings of spontaneous nystagmus, lateralization of the tuning fork to the well ear, and the possibility of otoscopic findings indicative of suppurative disease.

XIII. PHARYNGEAL BLEEDING

A. Bleeding from the mouth may be due to trauma but is most commonly observed following adenotonsillectomy or oral surgical procedures. Be alert to the possibility of an underlying hemorrhagic disorder. Secondary bleeding following adenotonsillectomy may occur at any time up to the twentieth postoperative day. The pulse rate and quality is a good indicator of the amount of bleeding, because an occasional vomiting of "coffee ground" material may represent but a small amount of the blood loss.

B. *Examination* is best conducted with the patient in the supine or head-low position and should include the nose, alveolar margins, floor of the mouth and the oro-, epi-, and hypopharynx. Topical anesthesia may be required in adults but should be used cautiously in children. General anesthesia, as a repeat performance, is dangerous and should be administered with caution and only when an adequate blood volume has been re-established.

C. Lacerations of the palate or pharynx may need to be sutured to control bleeding. Clots from the nasopharynx or tonsillar fossa may be removed by suction or with a gauze sponge stick. A bleeding point may be clamped and ligated. For generalized bleeding from an area, a sponge stick is used to apply a chemical cauterizing agent. If bleeding from the nasopharynx persists, a postnasal tampon is introduced. Blood replacement is an obvious requirement and so is hospitalization.

XIV. LARYNGEAL TRAUMA

A. Automobile accidents are responsible for most injuries in which the larynx is involved. The trauma usually occurs to the passenger in the front seat, whose extended neck strikes the dashboard. Direct laryngeal trauma may occur after a blow from a baseball bat or golf ball, a boxing injury, striking a protruding pipe or tree branch, garroting or the entanglement of a scarf or necktie in machinery.

B. SYMPTOMS AND DIAGNOSIS

Hoarseness, dysphonia or aphonia following a history of trauma is fairly indicative of some degree of soft tissue nerve or cartilaginous involvement of the larynx. *Respiratory* symptoms are: progressive stridor, dyspnea and suprasternal and infrasternal retractions and hemoptysis. Palpation of the neck in suspected laryngeal trauma may disclose subcutaneous emphysema, deformity and discoloration or fixation of the thyroid or cricoid cartilages or fracture of the hyoid bone. Often, the thyroid cartilage is flattened, or one ala is found to overlap the other anteriorly. Indirect laryngoscopy should always be attempted and may reveal hematoma, edema, vocal cord lacerations, deformity of the laryngeal configuration and impaired mobility of the vocal cords. The airway should always be evaluated at this time. Lateral and anteroposterior neck x-ray films for soft tissue detail may reveal air in the soft tissue spaces or deformity of the structures and should be ordered as soon as possible. Direct laryngoscopy and tracheoscopy are indicated in all cases of suspected laryngeal fracture. Early diagnosis and initiation of therapy are invaluable measures.

C. **TREATMENT**

The essence of therapy of laryngeal trauma is the maintenance and preservation of the airway. The extent of the injury serves as a guide. The treatment of minimal soft-tissue injury consists of external hot packs, voice rest, humidification and surveillance. If the airway is compromised, a low tracheotomy should be done before it becomes a desperate emergency. As soon as the patient's general condition will permit, fractured cartilages must be reduced, replaced and maintained in position. This may be done perorally or by open reduction. Failure or inadequate early management results in laryngeal stenosis and the need for a permanent tracheotomy.

XV. NASAL AND SINUS TRAUMA

A. The *historic elements* should include, in addition to events relevant to the local site of injury, an inquiry into lapses of consciousness, past history of nasofacial trauma either accidental or surgical, impairment of special sensory function (olfaction, vision, audition, equilibrium, phonation) and motor function (trismus, dysphagia, epiphora, extra-ocular immobility, etc.).

B. The *physical findings* are those of trauma and fractures in any area of the body—namely, pain, swelling, deformity and impairment of function. Appraise the vital functions of the patient, particularly the airway and cardiovascular system. Be alert for associated lesions—those apparent and in proximity to the trauma as well as those distant and perhaps occult (intrathoracic or intra-abdominal trauma, etc.).

C. Cerebrospinal fluid rhinorrhea (or otorrhea) is to be suspected whenever blood or secretion emanates from the nasal, oral or aural apertures. *X-ray films may include:*
   1. PA and right and left lateral projections of the nasal bones.

2. Upper occlusal view of the nasal arcade.
3. Waters projection to evaluate the maxillary sinuses, facial bones, orbit and mandible.
4. Submental vertex view to appraise the sphenoid sinuses, zygomatic arch and base of skull.
5. Caldwell projections to appraise the frontal and ethmoid sinuses.
6. Other specific x-ray projections may be obtained as need indicates.

D. MANAGEMENT

Treatment includes immediate measures to preserve and safeguard all tissues, even those severely traumatized and detached, active and/or passive immunization for tetanus prophylaxis, and final disposition of subsequent care of injured tissues and structures. At all times, the airway must be maintained.

CHAPTER 24

Ocular Emergencies

PETER C. KRONFELD, M.D.

I. INTRODUCTION

The ocular conditions which cause patients to present themselves in the Emergency Service of hospitals or clinics may vary greatly with regard to *urgency* and *seriousness* of the condition.

The following has proved useful in the management of large numbers of ocular emergencies.

A. Those conditions requiring immediate care:
    1. Severe chemical burns of conjunctiva or cornea.
    2. Large sharp foreign bodies "in the eye" (such as glass or splinters which, as a result of unavoidable lid or eye movements, may cause more trauma "by the minute").
    3. Occlusion of the central retinal artery or its branches.
    4. Acute angle-closure glaucoma.

B. Those necessitating symptomatic relief (because of intense photophobia, blepharospasm, foreign body sensation or pain):
    1. Certain forms of radiation or allergic conjunctivitis.
    2. Traumatic corneal abrasions.
    3. The usual small foreign bodies lodged in the corneal epithelium or in the upper tarsal conjunctiva.

C. Those demanding definitive therapy:
    1. Perforating or nonperforating injuries of the eyeball.
    2. Injuries to the surrounding structures.

D. Those of a contagious nature that must be recognized:

1. Epidemic keratoconjunctivitis.
2. Severe bacterial conjunctivitis.

E. Those needing recognition as not urgent, but requiring some reassurance and referral to the specialist:

A variety of ocular conditions which alarm the patient by the suddenness of onset or the conspicuousness—objective or subjective—of some of the symptoms.

II. IMMEDIATE CARE NEEDED

A. CHEMICAL BURNS OF CONJUNCTIVA OR CORNEA

1. The adoption of rigid safety measures (such as protective goggles) has reduced to an all-time low the number of chemical burns occurring in industry, in professional construction work and in chemical laboratories. Most burns now occur in the home, in private garages or hobby workshops, where amateurs work with tools and chemical agents with which they are not familiar. The offending agents are mostly detergents, window cleaning or other cleansing solutions and only rarely strong acids or strong bases.

2. Severely burned conjunctiva looks white and opaque and breaks down to shreds within a few hours; the cornea turns a dull white. Moderately damaged conjunctiva appears edematous and hyperemic.

3. Irrespective of the nature of the offending agent, first aid consists of copious irrigations of the conjunctival sac with water in the most readily available form. Tap water at room or body temperature makes an excellent irrigating fluid. Its use in a washbowl or sink in which the injured person can immerse the top of his head, including the burned eye, should be recommended over the telephone to any person reporting that such and such a fluid got into his or her eye. While the eye is under water, it is advisable to move the eyelids vigorously, if necessary with one's

fingers, so as to allow the water to penetrate into the recesses of the conjunctival sac.

4. In the Emergency Room of hospitals or clinics, again, it is most important that the condition be recognized promptly and treatment instituted immediately. To delay the irrigation until the "most suitable" fluid can be obtained from the pharmacy or until an irrigating tip can be sterilized would be a mistake. Sterile saline is preferable to unsterile saline, but tap water is preferable to any fluid that is not readily available. Large glass or plastic syringes with their own tips can serve as irrigators, but their limited capacity is a disadvantage. The following points are worth remembering.

    a. A few drops of a topical anesthetic (tetracaine, proparacaine or similar agent) instilled into the conjunctival sac facilitates the treatment for both patient and physician.

    b. The stream of fluid going in should be strong, that is, on the order of several milliliters per second.

    c. The spasm of the lid muscles elicited by the burn must be overcome by gentle pull on the eyelids (or, if necessary, with lid retractors).

    d. The tip of the irrigator should never touch the cornea.

    e. The recesses (fornices) of the conjunctival sac, particularly the upper one, should be kept in mind.

    f. The first irrigation should last about 10 minutes or, in a case of particulate foreign matter, until no more particles can be dissolved in the effluent.

5. Mild chemical burns not involving the cornea may not require more treatment than one irrigation, which, if justified by marked subjective discomfort, may be followed by instillations of a topical corticosteroid preparation every 3 or 4 hours for 1 or 2 days. A record of the patient's vision acuity

after the irrigation, with and without the pinhole disk,* can be of great medicolegal value. This also applies to the severely burned, who, usually and after a second irrigation half an hour later, have to be referred to an ophthalmologist for further care.

B. LARGE SHARP FOREIGN BODIES "IN THE EYE"

This category includes splinters of glass, plastic or metal measuring from 5-15 mm. in length whose sharp points or edges have cut into the eyeball in such a way as to give the foreign body an anchorage but still allow it to move with the movements of the lids of the eyeball. In these cases, the mere opening of the eye, voluntarily by the patient or manually by the examiner, can add severe additional trauma by pushing the foreign body more deeply into the eye. Where such situations are suggested by the history, it may be best to *delay examination* of the eye until the ophthalmologic consultant arrives and preparations for possible intraocular surgery have been made. First aid then consists of binocular eye dressings, a sedative-analgesic combination, a broad-spectrum antibiotic and physical immobilization of the patient.

C. OCCLUSION OF THE CENTRAL RETINAL ARTERY

1. The history is that of sudden pain and loss of vision in one eye. The objective findings are absence of the direct reaction of the pupil to light, diffuse gray edema of the retina and poor filling of the retinal vascular tree (as compared to that of the other eye). Since occlusion of the central retinal artery is a manifestation of systemic vascular disease, a physical examination should be done first. The prognosis with regard to return of vision depends on the duration and the degree of retinal anoxia. The former may be estimated from the history, the latter from

*The pinhole is a handy device for the approximate correction of refractive errors or other imperfections of the optical system.

the visual capacities of the eye in the state of anoxia. If the vision is limited to light perception in the temporal field and the duration is in excess of 4 hours, the chances of recovery are practically nil. If, on the other hand, the patient is seen within 2 hours of the onset of the condition and can count fingers at 2 or 3 feet, chances for a substantial return of vision are reasonably good.

2. First aid consists of measures aimed at elevation of the blood pressure plus vasodilation in the area supplied by the carotid arteries. Vigorous physical exercise for 3 to 5 minutes, alternating with breathing into a paper bag, is a widely used form of therapy. Vasodilation in the region of the ophthalmic artery may be produced by the retrobulbar injection of tolazoline hydrochloride (Priscoline), in doses of 25-50 mg. Beneficial effects on the intraocular circulation (in retina and choroid) are obtainable by making the eye hypotonic with acetazolamide (Diamox), in 500-mg. I.V. doses, plus withdrawal of the aqueous (paracentesis of the anterior chamber). The response, if any, starts immediately and continues for several hours and even days. If there is some immediate response, treatment with thrombolytic agents for 2-3 days offers a chance of further improvement.

D. ACUTE ANGLE-CLOSURE GLAUCOMA

1. Acute angle-closure glaucoma is a *true* ocular emergency; every hour of delay in recognition and treatment may mean (1) a definite amount of further visual loss and (2) poorer response to hypotensive therapy.

2. The diagnosis may be difficult in the not-too-infrequent cases in which the systemic symptoms overshadow the local disease. The vomiting, dehydration and subjective sensation of being extremely ill can lead the examiner astray unless he includes the eyes in his examination, which, in acute angle-closure glaucoma, show a characteristic picture of

(1) congestion, (2) steaminess of the cornea, (3) shallowness of the anterior chamber, (4) mydriasis and (5) a high tactile or tonometric tension. First aid should consist of a powerful, readily available miotic such as Eserine or pilocarpine in drop or ointment form (every 15 minutes in the case of drops and every half hour in the case of ointment, for the first 2 hours) aided by Diamox (500 mg. I.V.) and, if available, an osmotherapeutic agent (such as glycerin by mouth, 150-180 ml. of a 50% solution flavored with citrus fruit juice) or mannitol in doses of 1.5-2.0 Gm./kg. administered intravenously in a period of 30-60 minutes. Most acute attacks can thus be made to abate within about 6 hours, at which time an ophthalmologist should "take over."

III. SYMPTOMATIC RELIEF NEEDED

A. INTENSE OCULAR DISCOMFORT

1. Besides the large sharp foreign bodies referred to under II. B, there are less serious ocular conditions characterized by intense ocular discomfort with photophobia, blepharospasm or foreign body sensation dominating. Photophobia of a degree bordering on severe pain is the outstanding symptom of photophthalmias such as "snow blindness," welder's flash and related conditions. Phlyctenular keratoconjunctivitis, which is an acute allergic reaction to a product of the tubercle bacillus, can also be associated with intense photophobia.

2. First aid—in cases of photophthalmia—consists of instillations of epinephrine (0.1%) and cold applications. Only very rarely, and then only very sparingly, should topical anesthetics be used. Topical corticosteroid preparations have proved of great value in the treatment of allergic conjunctivitis. The adverse side effects of prolonged use of topical steroids (cataract, elevation of the intraocular pressure, increased pathogenicity of certain fungi and viruses) should be kept in mind.

3. Intense ocular discomfort with a history of minor trauma is usually due to a corneal abrasion.

B. CORNEAL ABRASION

1. The cornea is covered by a squamous stratified epithelium resting on a basement membrane. Objects brushing across the cornea, such as the edge of a sheet of stationery or a twig from a tree, can rub off portions of this epithelium and thereby cause a corneal abrasion (or erosion), which, by exposing sensory nerve endings, elicits photophobia, lacrimation, blepharospasm and an intense subjective sensation described by most patients as foreign body sensation rather than pain.

2. To the examiner, the objective and subjective symptoms may seem disproportionate to the size of the epithelial defect, which is often minute and demonstrable only by "staining" the cornea with fluorescein. This is most conveniently and safely done by gently touching the conjunctiva of the lower lid with the edge of one of the commercially available fluorescein paper strips. Only the exposed deeper layers of epithelium take the stain and turn green, in sharp contrast to the undamaged, and therefore unstained, surrounding surface layer of epithelium.

3. Except for the fortunately rare cases in which the epithelial defect becomes a portal of entry for bacterial or viral infections, corneal abrasions heal rapidly. Large doses of local anesthetics used topically for relief from the intense discomfort inhibit regeneration of epithelium and therefore delay the healing of the abrasion. Routine treatment aims at immobilization of the injured eye by a tightly applied eye dressing and an appropriate dose of a barbiturate, which helps the patient to get 8-12 hours of sound sleep. Twenty-four hours later, the eye should be re-examined. In most cases, the abrasion heals completely or almost completely within that time. In the rare cases of infection which are recognized by gray-to-yellow opaqueness of the floor of the defect,

identification of the invader and institution of the
appropriate anti-infective (antibacterial, antiviral,
antifungal) treatment are the essential steps for
which the patient should, with a minimum of delay,
be referred to an ophthalmologist. Frequent instillations of an antibiotic combination such as Neosporin
may serve as first aid and/or "temporary cover treatment."

C. THE USUAL SMALL FOREIGN BODY

1. Because of its exposed position and the receptacle-
    like construction of its lids, the human eye easily
    catches small airborne or mechanically propelled
    foreign bodies. The large majority, fortunately, do
    not carry much kinetic energy and are therefore
    stopped by the surface layer of cornea or conjunc-
    tiva. The movements of the eyeball and eyelids tend
    to press these foreign bodies slightly into the surface
    layer and thereby contribute to their "getting stuck,"
    which happens most frequently on the cornea and on
    the upper tarsal conjunctiva. They are removed from
    the latter with cotton-tipped applicators after ever-
    sion of the upper lid, which is accomplished most
    easily when the levator muscle is completely relaxed,
    as in extreme depression (downward rotation of the
    eye).
2. Foreign bodies are removed from the surface of the
    cornea with spud-like instruments under good topical
    anestheisa (3 to 4 instillations of anesthetics such as
    0.5% tetracaine or proparacaine). A good headrest
    and good focal illumination are essential require-
    ments. Most ophthalmologists remove corneal for-
    eign bodies under the conditions of illumination and
    magnification provided by the slit lamp. This meth-
    od can reduce greatly the amount of "digging," that
    is, disruption of normal tissue structure, necessary to
    introduce the instrument behind the foreign body.
3. In deciding whether a nonspecialist should undertake
    the removal of a corneal foreign body, one should

consider its location with regard to the center (optical portion) of the cornea. In any case, removal of a foreign body should be followed by instillation of a broad-spectrum antibiotic, application of a fairly tight eye dressing and, under any circumstances, reexamination of the eye 24 hours later.

IV. DEFINITIVE THERAPY NEEDED

A. INJURIES OF THE EYEBALL

1. The distinction between perforating and nonperforating injuries is of utmost importance. Perforating injuries entail the danger of (1) intraocular infection, (2) retention of a foreign body within the eyeball and (3) damage to the deeper, more delicate structures of the eye. The differentiation between perforating and nonperforating injuries is made on the basis of the eye findings, namely, a wound or portal of entry in the former and the signs of sudden stretching of the coats of the eyeball in the latter. The portal of entry can be very gross and unequivocal in some cases and almost microscopic in others. A careful analysis of the circumstances under which the accident occurred can yield invaluable clues.

2. First aid in perforating injuries consists of prophylactic anti-infective therapy. Because of the peculiar anatomic structure of the eye, it is *not* permissible to wait for definite signs of posttraumatic intraocular infection. Since bacteriologic findings usually are not available when the diagnosis of perforation is first made, the anti-infective treatment should be "all inclusive." Specific drug therapy is controversial and should be cleared by an ophthalmologist. The perforation may require plastic repair, which, as well as the removal of intraocular foreign bodies, will have to be left to the ophthalmologist. The recognition of the perforating character of the

injury and the initial dose of the anti-infective
agent may contribute more toward a favorable outcome than the most skillful plastic repair of the
wound performed by the ophthalmologist.

3. Blunt injuries (or contusions) of the eyeball are in-
flicted by relatively large, blunt, often round objects. During the impact, the eyeball wall is
stretched, which some of the ocular tissues (such as
the choroid) tolerate less well than others. In some
of these injuries, the mechanical stress is so great
that the eyeball wall actually ruptures.

4. In the more common milder cases, cornea and sclera
stretch sufficiently to allow for the deformation
caused by the injuring object, and intraocular hemorrhages of varying extent are the principal eye findings a few hours after injury. Treatment consists of
complete rest for several days to a week, since there
is a strong possibility of recurrence of the hemorrhage directly related to physical activity. The patient with a contused, partly blood-filled eye should,
therefore, be treated just like the patient with a
cerebral concussion or skull fracture.

B. INJURIES TO THE OCULAR ADNEXA

1. Lacerations of the eyelids are common and are generally considered emergencies. Before repairing these
   lacerations, three important points should be remembered:
   a. The eyeball should be carefully examined for
      signs of injury that may require surgical or medi-
      cal treatment by an ophthalmologist and that
      may be infinitely more important than the repair
      of the laceration.
   b. Lacerations including the lid border require more
      than the usual suturing in one or two layers if
      permanent notching of the border is to be
      avoided.
   c. Lacerations including the lower lacrimal canali-
      culus are difficult to repair and should therefore

be referred to surgeons with special experience in the field.

2. The typical fractures of orbital bones are (1) fracture, dislocation and/or comminution of the malar bone and (2) the "blowout" fracture of the floor of the orbit. These fractures are hardly emergencies, but should be suspected if the examination reveals definite downward displacement of the eye (with reference to the other eye) or diplopia in the upper field of gaze.

3. Extension of skull fractures into the optic canal is difficult to recognize even if the patient is sufficiently conscious to note the loss of vision. The management of the fracture should be left to the neurosurgeon.

V. CONTAGIOUS DISEASES

A. Some ocular diseases represent emergencies in the sense that prompt recognition and institution of therapy may prevent spread of the disease. A classic example is the so-called epidemic keratoconjunctivitis due to a well-defined virus which made its first large-scale appearance in the United States as shipyard conjunctivitis in 1942. The high communicability is due to the insensitivity of the virus to drying and dilution. No other agent has produced a comparable number of infections in physicians and nurses or a comparable degree of office and clinic epidemics.

B. The early symptoms may be much more impressive to the patient than to the physician. They are conjunctival and lid edema, especially of the caruncle and semilunar fold, with mild hyperemia and only scanty discharge in which mononuclear cells predominate, plus a definite swelling and tenderness of the preauricular gland. In any situations resembling this clinical picture, the most important consideration is prevention of spread of the disease. This may require a form of isolation which, in many households, may be difficult to accomplish.

C.   The occasional patient who presents himself in the
     Emergency Room with an acute or hyperacute bacterial
     conjunctivitis is readily recognized by the profuse mu-
     copurulent secretion exuding from his eye or eyes.
     Gram-stained conjunctival smears usually furnish enough
     clues with regard to the etiology and appropriate treat-
     ment. It is important to determine, at the first examina-
     tion, whether or not the patient's cornea is involved in
     the inflammatory disease.

VI. THE NONEMERGENCIES

A.   A good many visits to the Emergency Room are made
     by eye patients who are unable to contact an ophthal-
     mologist at the time of a sudden change in the condition
     of their eyes. No general rules apply to the management
     of such patients. An attempt, however, should be made
     to define and to record the condition in broad terms and
     then to steer the patient into the proper channels.

B.   A typical ophthalmologic nonemergency is the subcon-
     junctival hemorrhage that, because of its conspicuous-
     ness—a bright-red blotch against the white sclera—and
     also because of the apparent lack of a cause, tends to
     alarm the patient. The cause often is a minor, self-
     inflicted trauma (rubbing one's eyes during sleep) and
     the condition is only rarely an expression of a systemic
     vascular disease or of a blood dyscrasia.

CHAPTER 25

Allergic Emergencies

RAY F. BEERS, JR., M.D.

I. BRONCHIAL ASTHMA

A. Bronchial asthma is a common respiratory emergency.
The effective treatment of bronchospastic crisis requires that the following points be kept clearly in
mind:

1. *Sedation is rarely indicated.* Most sedatives tend to
depress the respiratory center and are potentially
dangerous. Morphine and its derivatives, as well as
morphine-like drugs (Meperidine, etc.), *must be entirely avoided,* unless the patient's ventilation is
completely under artificial control. In the rare instance of a highly frightened patient who is totally
unable to cooperate, ether in oil—1 part ether (0.5-
1.0 ml./kg.) to 2 parts of olive oil by rectum—combines prompt sedation with minimum risk.

2. *Antihistamine drugs are contraindicated in adult
asthma.* They are bronchoconstrictors, and some—
e.g., diphenhydramine (Benadryl) or promethazine
(Phenergan)—have anticholinergic side effects and
tend to decrease the flow of bronchial secretion,
which is *undesirable.*

3. *Aspirin should not be given to acute asthmatic patients* until the nature of the asthma is clearly established.

4. *Intravenous corticosteroids are not emergency
therapy.* Even though begun in the Emergency
Room, corticosteroid therapy will not produce appreciable effects for 3-6 hours.

5. *There are no reliable clinical signs of hypercarbia.*
When in doubt as to the need for artificial

ventilation, administer oxygen and determine the arterial P_{CO_2}. Normal Pa_{CO_2} is 35-45 mm. Hg. If prolonged artificial ventilation seems indicated, determine the arterial oxygen tension and pH as well. The 50-50 rule is helpful in determining the need for intensive care; i.e., if Pa_{O_2} is less than 50 mm. Hg and Pa_{CO_2} is greater than 50 mm. Hg, immediate transfer to the intensive respiratory care unit is indicated.

6. *Severe dyspnea and a quiet chest imply an ominous prognosis.* Wheezing (sibilant) rales depend on the movement of air through a narrowed bronchiole; if ventilation becomes inadequate, wheezing will cease despite the fact that the patient's condition is more grave.

7. *Effective treatment requires classification as to severity.* Consult the Table for a brief summary of workable criteria.

B. The criteria given in the Table must be modified in *children below age 2,* who show neither the positional preferences nor the anxiety of older children or adults with asthma. The severely asthmatic infant in this age group can lie comfortably, flat on his back and, even if cyanotic, will smile pleasantly when his attention is caught by a toy. *Tachypnea* is extremely pronounced in this age group and respiratory rates of 60-80 per minute are not uncommon. Respiratory movement is entirely abdominal and the chest, on auscultation, is often surprisingly quiet.

C. DRUGS FOR IMMEDIATE TREATMENT

1. *Epinephrine injection U.S.P. (epinephrine hydrochloride—1:1000).*—Dose: 0.01 mg./kg.—to a maximum of 0.30 mg. (0.30 ml.) or

    4 mo. - 1 yr.: 0.10 mg. (0.10 ml.)
    1 yr. - 2 yr.: 0.15 mg. (0.15 ml.)
    2 yr. - 3 yr.: 0.20 mg. (0.20 ml.)
    3 yr. - 6 yr.: 0.30 mg. (0.30 ml.)

SEVERITY OF ASTHMA

Criteria	Mild	Moderate	Severe	Extreme
Duration of wheezing	Less than 12 hr.	More than 12 but less than 24 hr.	Usually more than 24 hr.	Indeterminate
General appearance	Normal or excited; seldom true anxiety or fatigue	Normal or moderate anxiety; mild fatigue	Frightened; deep anxiety; very fatigued	Somnolescent, semicomatose or unconscious
Cough	Deep; produces some clear mucus	Repetitive, shallow cough; produces little expectoration	Unable to cough	Unable to cough
Posture	Prefers to sit, but can lie down	Semirecumbent posture possible	Cannot move from preferred position, i.e., sitting; thorax angled forward, elbows braced	Lies in any position; usually is placed semirecumbent
Respiratory chest excursion	Normal or increased	Normal or moderate decrease	Fixed in inspiration; no visible movement	No chest movement—shallow abdominal movements—at times, paradoxical
Color	Normal or somewhat red (hyperventilation)	Normal or subcyanotic	Ashen gray or deeply cyanotic	Deep cyanosis
Pulse rate	Normal or moderate tachycardia (100-120)—due to excitement	Moderate tachycardia, 120-140	Marked tachycardia, greater than 140	Rapid, thready pulse which may disappear entirely at times
Breath sounds (intensity)	Normal or increased	Normal or moderately decreased	Barely audible to absent	Usually absent
Rales	Numerous sibilant; many tubular	Mainly sibilant; occasional tubular	Occasional very high pitched, sibilant rales	Usually none
Response to epinephrine 0.30 mg. subcutaneously	Often dramatic and complete relief—rales may entirely disappear	Moderate relief; tubular rales now predominate	None or becomes worse	None or becomes worse
Pa_{O_2}	Normal	Normal	Less than 50 mm. Hg	Less than 50 mm. Hg
Pa_{CO_2}	Normal	Normal	Greater than 50 mm. Hg	Greater than 60 mm. Hg

The dose may be repeated at 20-minute intervals, provided improvement after each dose is apparent. If improvement does not occur after one or two doses, the drug should *not* be continued—*especially* in a child who does *not* expectorate. It is best to switch to aminophylline.

2. *Aminophylline U.S.P.—for I.V. administration* (10 ml. contains 250 mg.; 20 ml. ampule contains 500 mg.). Dose: 4 mg./kg./dose—not to exceed 15 mg./kg./24 hours. Administer slowly by syringe (1 ml. per minute). The initial injection may be followed by a slow (1-2 hour) I.V. infusion of the same or twice the amount in 250 ml., or more, of 5% glucose in water, if more prolonged therapy is necessary.

3. *Aminophylline for rectal administration (suppositories or solution).*—Various sizes are available; i.e., 125, 250, and 500 mg. Dose: 4-6 mg./kg./dose— not to exceed 30 mg./kg./24 hours. The individual dose should not be repeated in less than 4 to 6 hours.

4. *Isoproterenol hydrochloride inhalation U.S.P. (Isuprel—1:200) or epinephrine inhalation U.S.P. (1:100).*—Occasionally, mild-to-moderate bronchospasm will be dramatically relieved by two to three deep inhalations of these solutions nebulized from an appropriate hand-powered (DeVilbiss No. 40, Vaponephrine, etc.) or Freon-powered (Medihaler, Mistometer, etc.) nebulizer. At times, it is helpful to administer these drugs by means of an intermittent positive pressure breathing (IPPB) device. More commonly, these inhalations complete the relief that epinephrine injection has begun.

5. *Sodium bicarbonate (44.6 mEq.-50 ml.).*—Although this drug is more appropriately given in calculated increments to compensate respiratory acidosis when the blood pH is below 7.2 and the Pa_{CO_2} and Pao_2 are known, these measures are not always immediately available. In the moribund, or nearly moribund, asthmatic patient, respiratory acidosis can be

assumed and 1 (50 ml.) ampule, i.e., 44.6 mEq. given I.V., empirically to an adult, or 1 mEq./kilo to a child. If arterial blood pH is below 7.35, 2mEq./kilo can be given initially and repeated in 1-4 hours if acidosis persists as judged by arterial blood pH. Subsequent doses must be guided by the appropriate measures.

D. DRUGS FOR FOLLOW-UP CARE

Once the acute episode of bronchospasm has been relieved, there is, unfortunately, a strong tendency for the symptoms to recur within the next 24-72 hours. Adequate symptomatic medication during this period will prevent many repeat visits to the Emergency Room. Useful drugs are:

1. *Ephedrine sulfate, U.S.P.* – Dose: 0.5 mg./kg. – not to exceed 3 mg./kg./24 hours. A wide variety of tablets containing ephedrine sulfate, 25 mg. with a barbiturate (to minimize the CNS-stimulating effects of the ephedrine) are available (Amodrine, Tedral, Amesec, etc.). In children, it is often helpful to combine the dose of ephedrine in a sedative antihistamine-expectorant mixture (Phenergan Expectorant, Plain; Benylin Expectorant; etc.). Ephedrine, to a lesser degree, mimics the action of epinephrine; if expectoration is scanty, repeated doses must be used with caution.

2. *Potassium iodide.* – Dose: Three drops of saturated solution of potassium per year of age, to a maximum of 30-40 drops/24 hours is an effective expectorant. It should be given by mouth in 3-4 doses, with liberal amounts of fluid.

3. *Aminophylline for rectal administration.* – See C, 3. Given at 8-12-hour intervals, this agent is useful in preventing recurrence of bronchospasm, and can be used concomitantly with ephedrine and potassium iodide.

4. *Oral corticosteroids.* – An occasional brief (14-21 days) course of one of these drugs can be useful in preventing the need for hospitalization, should the

agents noted above fail to prevent repeated trips to
the Emergency Room. The dose of corticosteroids
is related to the severity of the symptoms, and the
size of the patient. Usually, an initial dose of 6 tablets per day (prednisone, 30 mg., triamcinolone, 24
mg., etc.) with gradual decrements (i.e., reducing by
1 tablet per day) to zero, is adequate.

E. OTHER DRUGS

1. *Intravenous corticosteroids.*—For the hospitalized
    patient in status asthmaticus, hydrocortisone sodium
    succinate, 50-100 mg. (or, in equivalent doses, pred-
    nisone-21-phosphate, dexamethasone phosphate,
    etc.) may be given and repeated in 2 hours and,
    thereafter, every 6 hours, as needed. In this situa-
    tion, the drug can be lifesaving.
2. *Sodium iodide.*—For expectorant purposes, the 10%
    solution can be added to an I.V. infusion containing
    aminophylline and a soluble steroid in the following
    doses:

Child	2.5 ml. (250 mg.)
Adolescent	5.0 ml. (500 mg.)
Adult	10.0 ml. (1 Gm.)

F. OTHER MEASURES

When the asthmatic patient is in extremis, the rapid insertion of an endotracheal tube coupled with artificial
ventilation by means of an IPPB device (Bird, Bennett,
Engstroem, etc.) and repeated tracheal lavage and suctioning may be life-saving. The anesthesia team should
be called. Developments over the next 24-72 hours will
decide whether a planned tracheotomy will be necessary.

II. ANAPHYLACTIC SHOCK

A. Anaphylactic (allergic) shock develops within seconds to
    minutes, usually after a parenteral injection given by
    medical personnel or a stinging insect. Insects sting any-
    where, but medical personnel should select sites which

permit the application of a tourniquet above the injection.

B. Occasionally, this state can follow the ingestion of *oral* agents, i.e., penicillin, quinidine, fish, cottonseed, etc. On extremely rare occasions, *inhalation*, i.e., penicillin, cottonseed, etc., may be responsible. The symptoms and signs occur in various combinations involving mainly four systems:

1. *Cardiovascular.* – Flushing and/or pallor; tachycardia and palpitation; blood pressure drop and/or complete circulatory collapse.

2. *Respiratory.* – Dyspnea (may be extreme), with or without wheezing; cyanosis (blue or gray); cough (repetitive) which may produce nothing, or frothy (at times blood-tinged) sputum.

3. *Cutaneous.* – Urticaria and/or angio-edema; itching (may be generalized or limited to the throat); and erythema (generalized or local).

4. *Gastrointestinal.* – Abdominal cramps (may be severe), followed by nausea, vomiting and diarrhea in various combinations. Itching, short cough and expiratory dyspnea, followed by cyanosis or pallor, shock and cessation of respiration (chest usually fixed in inspiration), might occur in rapid succession, and death is imminent unless immediate measures are taken.

C. **Treatment**

1. Apply a tourniquet above the injection site, if possible.

2. Give s.c., 1 mg. of epinephrine (1 ml. of epinephrine 1:1000)—0.50 ml. below the tourniquet and 0.50 ml. in the opposite arm (0.01 mg./kg. to a maximum of 0.50 mg. in the pediatric age group).

3. At the same time, *CALL FOR HELP.* This is a no. 1 emergency, and several pairs of hands are needed for all that must be done in a short period.

4. If shock is profound, it may be necessary to give 0.10 mg. of epinephrine I.V.; i.e., 0.10 ml. of the 1:1000 dilution mixed with 10 ml. of normal saline

(or the patient's blood)—given slowly. More rarely, the same dose can be given intracardially.

5. Ensure an adequate airway and give artificial respiration until oxygen can be administered under positive pressure by face mask or endotracheal catheter.

6. Find an adequate vein and place as large an indwelling needle (or venous cannula) as possible; if a vein cannot be found, cut down on a vein and cannulate—start an infusion of 1000 ml. of 5% glucose in water to keep the vein open for the addition of the following agents as the need arises.

7. Metaraminol bitartrate, U.S.P. (Aramine).—Available in 1 ml. ampules and 10 ml. vials—(10 mg./ml.). Can be given I.M. 3-25 mg. every 1-2 hours; as a single I.V. dose, 3-10 mg., or as a continuous I.V. infusion, 100-500 mg./liter, the drip rate depending on the blood pressure response.

8. Levarterenol bitartrate, U.S.P. (Levophed).—4 ml. ampules of the 0.2% solution (2 mg./ml.) are available. It can be given by *slow I.V. infusion only.* 8-16 mg. (4-8 ml., i.e., 1-2 ampules) added to 1000 ml. of 5% glucose in water, the drip rate being determined by the blood pressure response.

9. Aminophylline.—If bronchospasm, give 250-500 mg. of aminophylline (10-20 ml.)—VERY SLOWLY I.V.

10. *After adequate response,* I.V. antihistamines and/or corticosteroids might ensure continuing recovery and prevent relapse; since relapse is common, *the patient should be hospitalized* for continuing care.

11. Antihistamines and steroids are NOT emergency drugs.
    a. Diphenhydramine, U.S.P. (Benadryl)—25-50 mg. (1 mg./kg.); promethazine, U.S.P. (Phenergan)—12.5-25 mg. (0.5 mg./kg.); chlor- (Chlor-Trimeton) or brom- (Dimetane) pheniramine, U.S.P.—10 mg. (0.06 mg./kg.)—can be added to 250-1000 ml. of 5% glucose in water and given every 4 hours by slow I.V. drip.
    b. Hydrocortisone sodium succinate (Solu-Cortef)—100 mg. (or its equivalent)—I.V.

III. URTICARIA AND ANGIONEUROTIC EDEMA

A. Urticaria and angioneurotic edema are not medical emergencies unless the edema involves the larynx, where the sudden obstruction to the airway can prove fatal. Warning signs of this complication are:
   1. Itching of the palate and/or a feeling of fullness ("lump") in the throat.
   2. Voice change—hoarseness, etc.
   3. Cough and inspiratory stridor.
   4. Suprasternal notch and/or intercostal space retraction on inspiration. In infants, sternal retraction and/or paradoxic respiratory abdominal movement can be seen.

B. **Treatment**
   1. *Epinephrine injection, U.S.P.* (epinephrine hydrochloride—1:1000)—0.30 to 0.50 mg. (0.30 to 0.50 ml. of the 1:1000 dilution) subcutaneously and repeated in 10 to 20 minutes as necessary. Pediatric dose: 0.01 mg./kg. to a maximum of 0.50 mg.
   2. *25 mg. of diphenhydramine HCl* (Benadryl) or *promethazine HCl* (Phenergan) or 10 mg. chlor- (Chlor-Trimeton) or brom- (Dimetane) pheniramine, given I.M. or added to 250 ml. of 5% glucose in water and given by I.V. drip. Pediatric Doses: diphenhydramine U.S.P. (Benadryl)—1 mg./kg.; promethazine, U.S.P. (Phenergan)—0.5 ml./kg.; chlor- (Chlor-Trimeton) or brom- (Dimetane) pheniramine U.S.P.—0.06 mg./kg.
   3. *Patients with severe obstruction who do not respond* promptly to epinephrine and antihistamines may require tracheotomy.
   4. *Corticosteroids* act too slowly to be useful for the emergency treatment of acute angioneurotic edema.
   5. Urticaria without angio-edema of the larynx does not require epinephrine; in fact, it should be avoided because of possible "rebound" recurrence of symptoms. Patients with massive generalized urticaria might fail to obtain relief from oral antihistamines, but will respond if antihistamines are given intravenously.

6. *Follow-up care.* —"Around-the-clock" antihistamines by mouth for the next 3-4 days to prevent recurrence, e.g.:
   a. Chlorpheniramine (Chlor-Trimeton, Teldrin)—12 mg., t.i.d. p.c.
   b. Diphenhydramine (Benadryl)—25-50 mg., or promethazine (phenergan)—25-50 mg., h.s.

IV. SERUM SICKNESS (INCLUDING ANTITOXIN AND DELAYED PENICILLIN REACTIONS)

A. Although urticaria is a prominent component of serum-type reactions, any organ system may be affected. The patient should be carefully checked for:

Fever

Petechiae

Hematuria (microscopic)

Lymphadenopathy

Joint swelling

Friction rubs (pleural and pericardial)

Hepatomegaly

Evidence of peripheral neuritis (especially brachial plexus)

Evidence of Guillain-Barré syndrome

B. If none of these signs or symptoms is present, the treatment is the same as for any other urticaria. If one or more of the above symptoms and signs are present, prolonged treatment, probably requiring systemic corticosteroids, is indicated—and the patient should be hospitalized.

V. EXFOLIATIVE DERMATITIS

Exfoliative dermatitis is a serious generalized disease requiring hospitalization. Emergency Room treatment is NOT required.

CHAPTER 26

Proctologic Emergencies

JOSEPH P. CANNON, M.D., F.A.C.S.

I. INTRODUCTION

Every Emergency Service should have available an anoscope and a regular 25-cm. sigmoidoscope with a reliable light source. An aspirating machine providing adequate suction is necessary to remove feces, blood or pus. An electrocoagulation device should be available for emergency rectal hemostasis and incision and draining procedures. A large 30-cm. metal aspirating tube is also required.

II. FECAL IMPACTIONS

A. HISTORY

1. Change in bowel habits.
2. Feeling of constant rectal pressure.
3. As a rule, the patient has been taking antidiarrheal medication; i.e., paregoric, Lomotil, etc.
4. Generally found in the elderly and/or debilitated groups or tense nervous children and young adults.

B. OBJECTIVE FINDINGS

1. Adequate digital examination will palpate a large, rock-like fecal bolus with soft stool oozing around the mass.
2. If no mass is palpable, have the patient strain as if defecating and the mass will be palpable to index finger.
3. In rare cases a large mass will be revealed in the sigmoid on sigmoidoscopy.

405

C. TREATMENT

1. Removal of fecaloma with patient in knee-chest position.
2. Soft rubber 20-25 French catheter is inserted and guided past the rectal mass with index finger.
3. Two Fleet oil retention enemas are given and retained as long as possible.
4. Patient is re-examined and if lower bowel is clear, sigmoidoscopy is done at this time.
5. If mass is not passed, digital manipulation will aid in breaking it up for evacuation.
6. If patient is in severe pain:
   a. Inject 2-5 cc. of 1% Xylocaine into each quadrant of rectal sphincter.
   b. Use caudal block—but stand clear!
7. Follow-up treatment:
   a. Instruct the patient to drink more fluids.
   b. Increase bulk of the stool with more vegetables and fruit.
   c. Take a bulk laxative such as Hydrocil Fortified.

III. PERIRECTAL ABSCESS

A. HISTORY

1. Can occur in any age group but is rare in children.
2. The patient complains of rectal pain, pressure, inability to sit and chills and fever for 24-48 hours.

B. OBJECTIVE FINDINGS

1. Erythema with fluctuation in perianal area.
2. If (1) is not present, do anoscopy to visualize an infected anal crypt which will be oozing from the involved area.
3. If above are not found, have the patient take sitz baths every 4 hours and re-examine frequently.

C. TREATMENT

1. Using 1% Xylocaine with epinephrine, inject intra-
    dermally (pig skin) over the abscess. (If the needle
    goes deeper, the pressure in the abscess increases
    and so does the pain.)
2. Allow adequate time (5 minutes) for anesthesia to
    take effect and supplement if necessary.
3. Use electrocautery on cutting current to open
    abscess *widely*.
4. Use hemostats to open undermined tracts.
5. Use electrocautery on coagulation to control bleed-
    ers.
6. Have patient put ice packs over incision for 24
    hours.
7. Start constant warm wet compresses during the day
    after the first 24 hours.
8. Treat the wound weekly with 10% silver nitrate,
    neutralized with 1:1000 tincture of Zephiran.
9. Warn patient that this will probably develop into a
    fistula-in-ano and require further surgery.
10. Do gram stain, culture and sensitivities.
11. Prescribe antibiotics on basis of gram stain and cul-
    ture when available.

IV. ACUTE FISSURE IN ANO

A. HISTORY AND SYMPTOMS

Acute rectal pain during and following defecation
(diarrhea or constipation) which may last several minutes to many hours. Traces of bleeding may be found
on toilet tissue.

B. OBJECTIVE FINDINGS

1. Rectal spasm which increases when buttocks are
    held under tension.

2. An inverted V-shaped tag with a fiery raw base. Bleeding is not noted on this examination.
3. Anoscopic examination causes extreme pain and visualizes the raw area posteriorly with small hypertrophic anal papillae.

C. TREATMENT

1. Cauterization of anal fissure with 10% silver nitrate on applicator, then neutralized with 1:1000 tincture of Zephiran.
2. Patient to use Tucks pads for cleansing following defecation and at bedtime.
3. Dilation of rectum with finger cot following cleansing with ointment.
   a. Hydrocortisone 0.5%, Bacitracin ointment, 10 Gm., Neobase q.s. ad 30 Gm. or
   b. Gadoment ointment.
4. Sitz baths for 20 minutes every 4 hours if possible—comfortably warm, not hot.
5. Advise patient that if gradual improvement is not obtained in 3 weeks (approximately), surgery may be recommended.
6. Bulk laxative, e.g., Hydrocil Fortified, is advised—2 teaspoons at bedtime.

VI. INFECTED PILONIDAL CYST

A. HISTORY AND SYMPTOMS

1. Patient born with defect. Complains of pain, aggravated by sitting.
2. Usually found in overweight, hairy, teen-age males.

B. TREATMENT

Same as for perirectal abscess.

VII. ACUTE THROMBOTIC HEMORRHOIDS

A. HISTORY AND SYMPTOMS

1. Sudden onset of pain followed by a palpable rectal mass.
2. Not related to patient's activity but frequently occurs during defecation.

B. OBJECTIVE FINDINGS

1. Purple mass is present at mucocutaneous line of rectum.
2. Painful to touch and nonreducible.

C. TREATMENT

1. Infiltration of hemorrhoid and sphincter with 1% Xylocaine.
2. Elliptica excision of overlying skin and evacuation of clot.
3. Hemostasis with:
   a. Silver nitrate, (either sticks or a 10% solution) neutralized with 1:1000 tincture of Zephiran.
   b. Electrocoagulation.
   c. Catgut 2-0 sutures.
4. After care:
   a. Ice bag for 24 hours.
   b. Sitz baths, 4 times daily for 20 minutes each time.
   c. Follow weekly postoperatively.

VIII. RECTAL PROLAPSE

A. HISTORY AND SYMPTOMS

1. Condition generally found in elderly but has been seen in patients in their 30s.
2. Large painful mass felt by patient as a rule after straining at defecation or severe coughing.
3. Patient unable to replace "hemorrhoids."

B. OBJECTIVE FINDINGS

1. Large purplish circumferential mass protruding 2-12 cm. from anus with extreme rectal spasm and pain.
2. If patient has not sought medical aid, changes of impending gangrene (black with oozing of bright blood) are noted.

C. TREATMENT

1. *Early cases:* Knee chest position, attempt to reduce edema by *gentle* digital pressure. If not successful, inject 1% Xylocaine into rectal sphincter and replace prolapse manually. Apply pressure dressing, then tape buttocks.
2. *Late cases:* Constant warm wet compresses. Do not reduce manually because of danger of pelvic emboli and sepsis. Allow gangrenous tissue to demarcate with the aid of antibiotics before any surgery is considered.

IX. FOREIGN BODIES

A. HISTORY AND SYMPTOMS

1. Pain and/or feeling of pressure; usually history of ingestion of alcohol in large amounts.
2. *Ingested:* Bones (chicken, rib, etc.) are frequently found wedged in rectum.
3. *Self-administered:* Large objects such as water glasses, beer bottles, wire coat hangers, vibrating devices, cucumbers, etc.

B. TREATMENT

1. Removal under anesthesia if necessary. *Always* do sigmoidoscopy after removal to note bleeding and possible perforation. *Always* check, postremoval, with upright abdomen film for free air.

X. RECTAL HEMORRHAGE

A. HISTORY AND SYMPTOMS

Sudden onset of rectal bleeding varying from bright red to maroon in color. Can occur in any age group.

B. OBJECTIVE FINDINGS

Bright to dark blood in rectal vault.

C. TREATMENT

1. Digital and anoscopic examination to rule out internal hemorrhoids.
2. Sigmoidoscopy to rule out polyps, ulcerative colitis and low malignancies.
3. If above negative, have patient squat and strain. A bleeding internal hemorrhoid can be seen readily.
4. If above negative, emergency barium enema should be done.
5. If barium enema is negative, an upper G.I. series and small bowel series should be done.

All of these problems are painful, as is their treatment. Medications such as Darvon Compound 65 mg., Empirin #3 and Phenaphen with codeine, 30 mg., should be given freely, bearing in mind that codeine is constipating.

Index